T0330979

IN THE NAME OF PROGRESS
The Dark Side of Medical Research

IN THE NAME OF PROGRESS
The Dark Side of Medical Research

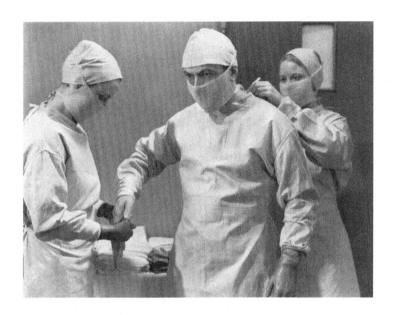

Campion Quinn, MD
Rockville Medical, LLC, USA

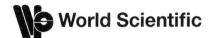

World Scientific

EW JERSEY · LONDON · SINGAPORE · BEIJING · SHANGHAI · HONG KONG · TAIPEI · CHENNAI · TOKYO

Published by

World Scientific Publishing Co. Pte. Ltd.

5 Toh Tuck Link, Singapore 596224

USA office: 27 Warren Street, Suite 401-402, Hackensack, NJ 07601

UK office: 57 Shelton Street, Covent Garden, London WC2H 9HE

Library of Congress Control Number: 2024024454

British Library Cataloguing-in-Publication Data
A catalogue record for this book is available from the British Library.

IN THE NAME OF PROGRESS
The Dark Side of Medical Research

ISBN 978-981-12-9181-4 (hardcover)
ISBN 978-981-12-9182-1 (ebook for institutions)
ISBN 978-981-12-9183-8 (ebook for individuals)

For any available supplementary material, please visit
https://www.worldscientific.com/worldscibooks/10.1142/13802#t=suppl

Desk Editors: Aanand Jayaraman/Joy Quek

Typeset by Stallion Press
Email: enquiries@stallionpress.com

Printed in Singapore

This book is devoted to Dr. Samir Patel, whose remarkable journey as a physician, entrepreneur, and philanthropist continues to inspire. His unwavering dedication to advancing healthcare, coupled with his entrepreneurial spirit and philanthropic endeavors, has left an indelible mark on the world. I call him my friend with great pride and profound respect.

About the Author

Campion Quinn, MD, FACP, MHA, is a distinguished physician, author, and medical consultant with over 20 years of clinical experience. Board-certified in internal medicine, emergency medicine, and geriatric medicine, Dr. Quinn also holds a Master of Healthcare Administration. As a clinician and associate clinical professor of medicine at the State University of New York, he has contributed significantly to the fields of clinical diagnosis, treatment, and medical management.

Dr. Quinn's career is marked by a strong commitment to advocacy and education, which is evident in his roles as medical director and chief medical officer for various healthcare organizations. His collaborations with key opinion leaders and pharmaceutical companies have led to notable advancements in medical therapies. His extensive body of work includes numerous journal articles and medical texts, with recent publications focusing on the ethical challenges in medical research.

In the Name of Progress: The Dark Side of Medical Research, Dr. Quinn illuminates the dark side of medical advancements, offering a comprehensive and candid exploration of historical and contemporary abuses. This book is a testament to his dedication to ethical medical practices and patient advocacy.

Contents

Introduction

The history of medical experimentation is a complex and often troubling narrative. While pursuing medical knowledge has led to countless advancements that have saved lives and alleviated suffering, it has also been marred by episodes of profound ethical violations. This book aims to explore the darker side of medical research, where patients were exploited, deceived, and subjected to inhumane treatments in the name of science.

From the early 20th century to the present day, various infamous experiments have highlighted the ethical breaches that can occur when scientific curiosity is unchecked by moral considerations. The Guatemala experiments and the Tuskegee syphilis study are stark reminders of how racial prejudice and the dehumanization of certain groups can lead to gross injustices. Similarly, the MK-Ultra and Montreal experiments showcase the extent to which governmental and institutional secrecy can facilitate the abuse of vulnerable individuals under the guise of national security.

In examining the SUPPORT trial, the Willowbrook experiments, and the Fernald experiments, we see how institutionalized settings, such as hospitals and schools, can become arenas for unethical research when oversight is inadequate. The story of Henrietta Lacks, whose cells were taken without her consent and used for decades in research, underscores the ongoing issues of consent and the exploitation of marginalized communities in medical research.

Each chapter delves into a specific case, providing a detailed account of the experiments, the researchers involved, and the victims. We explore the ethical violations and the long-term impacts on the individuals and communities affected. Importantly, this book also tracks the regulatory changes these abuses have spurred, illustrating how these dark chapters in medical history have led to stricter ethical guidelines and protections for research subjects.

To maintain the credibility and reliability of the information presented, all claims are meticulously substantiated with citations from reputable sources. Where there are gaps in knowledge, these are openly acknowledged. The language used is clear and direct, avoiding unnecessary technical jargon to ensure accessibility for all readers. Practical examples and varied sentence structures keep the material engaging and easy to follow.

In writing this book, I aim to shed light on these historical abuses, remember and honor the victims, and educate and inform current and future healthcare professionals, researchers, and the general public. By understanding the past, we can better safeguard the ethics of medical research in the future and ensure that the pursuit of knowledge never again comes at such a high human cost.

Chapter 1

Introduction to Medical Research Ethics

"The men's status did not warrant ethical debate. They were subjects, not patients; clinical material, not sick people."

— Allan M. Brandt,
"Racism and Research: The Case of the Tuskegee
Syphilis Study" (1978).[1]

In the annals of medical research, the pursuit of knowledge has often been marred by a troubling disregard for the sanctity of human life and dignity. The chilling observation by Allan Brandt at the beginning of this chapter serves as a blatant reminder of the dark chapters in medical history, where the zeal for scientific advancement eclipsed the fundamental principles of humanity and ethics. As we delve into the complex and often harrowing world of medical research ethics, it is imperative to confront these uncomfortable truths. We must scrutinize the past to understand how the noble field of medicine has, at times, been complicit in acts that betrayed the very essence of its Hippocratic oath. This chapter aims not only to shed light on the historical perspective of patient rights and informed consent but also to underscore the critical role of physicians and researchers in upholding the highest ethical standards in their quest for medical breakthroughs.

---

[1] Brandt, A.M. (1978). Racism and research: The case of the Tuskegee Syphilis study. *The Hastings Center Report.* 8(6):21–29.

1

Introduction to Ethical Principles in Medical Research

At the heart of medical research lies a complex interplay of scientific inquiry and ethical considerations. Ethics in medical research refers to the set of moral principles that guide researchers in the conduct of experiments and clinical trials. These principles are essential in ensuring that the dignity, rights, and welfare of research participants are respected and protected.

The importance of ethics in medical research cannot be overstated. It serves as a compass that guides researchers in making morally sound decisions, particularly when faced with dilemmas where the pursuit of scientific knowledge may conflict with the rights of individuals. Ethical research practices are crucial for maintaining public trust in the medical research community. They ensure that the research conducted not only adheres to the highest standards of scientific integrity but also respects and safeguards the well-being of participants.

Ethical considerations in medical research encompass a broad spectrum of issues, including but not limited to informed consent, confidentiality, risk–benefit analysis, and the equitable selection of research subjects. The fundamental ethical principles that underpin these considerations include the following:

- **Respect for Autonomy**: Acknowledging and respecting the decision-making capabilities of participants. This involves providing adequate information about the research and ensuring that consent is obtained freely without coercion. Further, that consent can be revoked at any time by the patient.
- **Beneficence:** The principle of doing good, ensuring that the research is conducted with the intent of bringing about a positive impact, such as advancing scientific understanding or improving healthcare outcomes.
- **Non-maleficence:** A commitment to avoid causing harm. Researchers are obligated to minimize risks and prevent harm to participants.
- **Justice:** Ensuring fairness in the distribution of the benefits and burdens of research. This principle demands that individuals or groups are not unfairly included or excluded from participation in research.

The evolution of these ethical principles has been shaped significantly by historical events in medical research, leading to the establishment of various codes and regulations. These principles not only guide researchers in conducting ethical research but also form the basis of regulatory frameworks that govern research practices globally.

Historical Perspective on Patient Rights and Informed Consent

The journey of medical research through history is marked by periods where the absence of formal guidelines led to profound ethical breaches. In the nascent stages of medical experimentation, the rights of patients were often overlooked, and the concept of informed consent was largely unrecognized. This era, characterized by a lack of regulatory oversight, saw researchers pursuing scientific discovery with little regard for the implications for their human subjects.

One of the most infamous examples from this period is the Thalidomide tragedy of the late 1950s and early 1960s. Thalidomide, initially marketed as a safe sedative for pregnant women to combat morning sickness, led to catastrophic birth defects in thousands of babies. This tragedy underscored the dire consequences of inadequate drug testing and the lack of informed consent, as the risks were not fully communicated to the patients.

Similarly, the Willowbrook Hepatitis experiments, conducted from 1956 to 1970, involved the deliberate infection of intellectually disabled children with hepatitis virus at the Willowbrook State School in New York. These experiments were rationalized under the pretext of studying the natural history of infectious diseases and developing a vaccine. However, the ethical implications of intentionally infecting vulnerable children, who could not provide informed consent, were largely ignored.

These events, along with the Tuskegee Syphilis Study, where African American men were denied treatment for syphilis, and the horrific human experiments conducted during the Nazi regime, highlight the urgent need for ethical reform in medical research. The Nuremberg Code of 1947,[2]

---

[2] https://research.unc.edu/human-research-ethics/resources/ccm3_019064/#:
~:text=The%20Nuremberg%20Military%20Tribunal's%20decision,medical%20
experimentation%20on%20human%20subjects (Accessed 1/28/24).

emerging from the trials of war criminals, was one of the first documents to articulate the necessity of voluntary consent in human experimentation. The Nuremberg Code, drafted at the end of the Nazi Doctor's trial in Nuremberg, has been hailed as a landmark document in medical and research ethics. Close examination of this code reveals that it was based on the Guidelines for Human Experimentation of 1931.[3] The 10 points of the code are as follows:[4]

1. The voluntary consent of the human subject is absolutely essential. This means that the person involved should have legal capacity to give consent; should be so situated as to be able to exercise free power of choice, without the intervention of any element of force, fraud, deceit, duress, overreaching, or other ulterior form of constraint or coercion; and should have sufficient knowledge and comprehension of the elements of the subject matter involved as to enable him to make an understanding and enlightened decision. This latter element requires that before the acceptance of an affirmative decision by the experimental subject there should be made known to him the nature, duration, and purpose of the experiment; the method and means by which it is to be conducted; all inconveniences and hazards reasonably to be expected; and the effects upon his health or person which may possibly come from his participation in the experiment. The duty and responsibility for ascertaining the quality of the consent rests upon each individual who initiates, directs, or engages in the experiment. It is a personal duty and responsibility which may not be delegated to another with impunity (see footnote 4).

2. The experiment should be such as to yield fruitful results for the good of society, unprocurable by other methods or means of study, and not random and unnecessary in nature.

3. The experiment should be so designed and based on the results of animal experimentation and a knowledge of the natural history of the

[3] Ghooi, R.B. (2011). The Nuremberg Code-A critique. *Perspect Clin Res.* 2(2):72–76. doi: 10.4103/2229-3485.80371.

[4] Nuremberg Code. *The Doctor's Trial: The Medical Case of the Subsequent Nuremberg Proceedings.* United States Holocaust Memorial Museum Online Exhibitions (Accessed 2/19/24).

disease or other problem under study that the anticipated results will justify the performance of the experiment.

4. The experiment should be so conducted as to avoid all unnecessary physical and mental suffering and injury.

5. No experiment should be conducted where there is an *a priori* reason to believe that death or disabling injury will occur, except, perhaps, in those experiments where the experimental physicians also serve as subjects.

6. The degree of risk to be taken should never exceed that determined by the humanitarian importance of the problem to be solved by the experiment.

7. Proper preparations should be made, and adequate facilities provided to protect the experimental subject against even remote possibilities of injury, disability, or death.

8. The experiment should be conducted only by scientifically qualified persons. The highest degree of skill and care should be required through all stages of the experiment of those who conduct or engage in the experiment.

9. During the course of the experiment, the human subject should be at liberty to bring the experiment to an end if he has reached the physical or mental state where continuation of the experiment seems to him to be impossible.

10. During the course of the experiment, the scientist in charge must be prepared to terminate the experiment at any stage, if he has probable cause to believe, in the exercise of the good faith, superior skill, and careful judgment required of him that a continuation of the experiment is likely to result in injury, disability, or death to the experimental subject.

This code laid the groundwork for the Declaration of Helsinki in 1964,[5] which provided a comprehensive framework emphasizing the balance between research benefits and ethical considerations.

---

[5] https://www.wma.net/policies-post/wma-declaration-of-helsinki-ethical-principles-for-medical-research-involving-human-subjects/ (Accessed 1/28/24).

The evolution of ethical standards in medical research, catalyzed by these tragedies, marked a pivotal shift toward prioritizing patient rights and informed consent. These historical instances serve as a stark reminder of the critical importance of ethical considerations in medical research, shaping the contemporary landscape, where the welfare of research subjects is paramount.

The Development of Informed Consent: From the Declaration of Helsinki to the Belmont Report

"In medical research involving human subjects, the well-being of the individual research subject must take precedence over all other interests." (see footnote 5).

— Declaration of Helsinki, World Medical Association.

The evolution of informed consent in medical research is a narrative of progressive ethical awakening, shaped significantly by historical missteps. The Declaration of Helsinki, established in 1964 by the World Medical Association, marked a pivotal moment in this journey. The Declaration of Helsinki is a seminal document in the field of medical ethics, guiding physicians and other participants in medical research involving human subjects. It was created in response to the growing awareness of the need for stringent ethical standards in the wake of atrocities like the Nazi experiments. It represents a cornerstone ethical code, setting forth principles to ensure respect for individuals and safeguarding their health and rights during research. Key tenets include the necessity of obtaining informed consent, the importance of ensuring participant welfare, the requirement for scientifically and ethically valid research protocols, and the mandate for independent committee review of research. The Declaration emphasizes that the well-being of research participants should always take precedence over the interests of science and society. As a globally recognized standard, it has profoundly influenced ethical guidelines and legislation worldwide, shaping the conduct of medical research and reinforcing the commitment to ethical principles in the pursuit of scientific knowledge.

The Belmont Report

"Respect for persons demands that subjects enter into the research voluntarily and with adequate information."

— The Belmont Report, National Commission for the Protection of Human Subjects of Biomedical and Behavioral Research.[6]

The Belmont Report (see footnote 6) of 1979 was developed in response to the public outcry over the Tuskegee Syphilis Study. It builds on the principles outlined in the Declaration of Helsinki and is a foundational document in the ethics of human subject research in the United States. It provides a comprehensive framework for understanding informed consent. The Report defines informed consent through three core components:

- **Information:** The Belmont Report emphasizes that individuals should be provided with sufficient information to make an informed decision about their participation in research. This information includes details about the research purpose, procedures, risks and benefits, alternatives to participation, and the right to withdraw from the research at any time.
- **Comprehension:** The report recognizes that merely providing information is not enough; the potential subject must also understand it. This understanding depends on the manner and context in which the information is conveyed and the cognitive and language proficiency of the participant. Researchers are responsible for ensuring that the participant comprehends the information, which may involve adapting the communication method to the individual's needs.
- **Voluntariness:** Informed consent must be given voluntarily, free from coercion, undue influence, or manipulation. The Belmont Report underscores the importance of the participant's freedom to decide without being subjected to any form of pressure or coercion by the researcher or others.

---

[6] https://www.hhs.gov/ohrp/regulations-and-policy/belmont-report/index.html (Accessed 1/28/24).

The Belmont Report's definition of informed consent is grounded in the principle of respect for persons, which entails treating individuals as autonomous agents capable of making their own decisions, while also protecting those with diminished autonomy. This definition has profoundly influenced research ethics, guiding the development of informed consent processes in research involving human subjects.

The Belmont Report's emphasis on informed consent was revolutionary. It mandated that participants must be given comprehensive information about the research, including its purpose, duration, procedures, risks, benefits, and alternative treatments. Furthermore, it asserted the necessity of ensuring that this consent is given voluntarily, without any form of coercion or undue influence, and with the provision for participants to withdraw at any time.

The shadow of historical abuses in medical research looms large over contemporary ethical practices. These events have been instrumental in shaping current attitudes and regulations concerning patient rights and research methodologies. The ethical breaches of the past have instilled a heightened sense of responsibility within the medical research community, leading to the establishment of rigorous ethical review processes.

Today, Institutional Review Boards (IRBs) or Ethics Committees are a standard part of any research involving human subjects. An IRB is a committee that reviews research methods involving human subjects. IRBs are also known as ethical review boards, research ethics boards, or independent ethics committees.

IRBs are responsible for the following:

- ensuring that research projects are ethical,
- protecting the rights and welfare of research participants,
- ensuring that research complies with regulations, ethical standards, and institutional policies,
- providing oversight of research.

IRBs are usually located at the site of the research study. They can approve, require modifications, or disapprove research. If an IRB approves a conditional approval, the IRB will require changes to be presented in writing and approved.

IRBs are legally required in some countries in certain circumstances. In the United States, research institutions can extend federal regulatory requirements to all of their human-subject research. Research conducted outside of the United States but funded by the US government is also subject to the same federal regulations.

IRBs include at least one member who is not affiliated with the institution and one member who is not a scientist. The IRB also has consultants who advise the board and are periodically involved in protocol review.

In short, IRBs are tasked with ensuring that all research proposals comply with ethical standards, including informed consent. The legacy of past abuses has also led to greater public awareness and scrutiny of medical research, fostering an environment where transparency and accountability are paramount.

Moreover, the impact of these historical events extends to the global stage, influencing international guidelines and policies. The principles outlined in the Declaration of Helsinki and the Belmont Report have been integrated into numerous international regulations and codes of conduct, guiding ethical medical research across the world.

The development of informed consent from the Declaration of Helsinki to the Belmont Report, and the lessons learned from historical abuses, have been fundamental in shaping modern research ethics. They serve as a constant reminder of the importance of respecting and protecting human subjects in medical research, ensuring that the dark chapters of the past are not repeated.

The Role of Physicians and Researchers in Upholding Ethical Standards

Physicians and researchers in the medical field are entrusted with a unique and dual responsibility: the provision of patient care and the advancement of medical research. This dual role is underpinned by a commitment to uphold stringent ethical standards, ensuring that the pursuit of scientific knowledge does not compromise patient welfare.

In patient care, physicians are guided by the Hippocratic injunction of "primum non nocere."[7] This is a Latin phrase that translates as "first, do no harm." This tenet demands that any treatment or care provided must prioritize the patient's health and well-being. In the context of research, this principle extends to ensuring that the rights, safety, and well-being of research participants are safeguarded throughout the study process. Physicians and researchers must navigate this landscape with a keen awareness of the potential ethical dilemmas that can arise from balancing patient care with research objectives.

The advancement of medical research often involves exploring uncharted territories and pushing the boundaries of scientific knowledge. While this pursuit is vital for medical progress, it must be conducted with an unwavering commitment to ethical principles. Researchers are responsible for designing and conducting studies that are scientifically sound and ethically justified. This involves ensuring that studies are necessary, that risks to participants are minimized and justified by the potential benefits, and that participants are selected fairly and without bias.

A critical aspect of upholding ethical standards in research is informed consent.[8] Researchers must ensure that participants are fully informed about the nature of the study, including any potential risks and benefits, and that they voluntarily agree to participate without coercion. This process is not merely a bureaucratic step but a fundamental expression of respect for the autonomy and dignity of participants.

Moreover, physicians and researchers must be vigilant against conflicts of interest that could compromise their judgment or the integrity of the research. Physicians and biomedical researchers often collaborate with pharmaceutical, medical device, and biotechnology companies. These partnerships are common and have led to significant advancements, especially in creating new medical tests and treatments. However, these collaborations also pose risks. There's a concern that the industry's financial objectives might clash with the medical profession's goals, potentially

---

[7]Gifford, R.W. (1977). Primum Non Nocere. *JAMA*. 238(7):589–590. doi:10.1001/jama. 1977.03280070029018.

[8]https://www.hhs.gov/ohrp/regulations-and-policy/guidance/faq/informed-consent/index. html (Accessed 1/28/24).

leading to conflicts of interest. Therefore, they are obliged to disclose any potential conflicts and take steps to mitigate them, ensuring that their primary allegiance remains with the welfare of patients and research participants.[9]

The role of physicians and researchers in upholding ethical standards in medical research is multifaceted and critical. It requires a delicate balance between patient care and the pursuit of scientific advancement, guided by a commitment to respect, beneficence, and justice. As guardians of ethical research, they play a pivotal role in maintaining public trust in the medical research community and ensuring that the legacy of medical research is defined not just by scientific achievements but also by its adherence to the highest ethical standards.

Navigating Conflicts of Interest

Conflicts of interest in medical research can significantly challenge the integrity of research and the trust placed in the medical community. These conflicts arise when a researcher's personal or financial interests potentially influence their professional judgment and responsibilities. A vivid example is the case of the antidepressant Paxil, where studies funded by the manufacturer initially downplayed the risk of suicide in adolescents. Later independent reviews highlighted these risks, leading to legal actions and changes in prescribing information.[10]

To navigate these conflicts, transparency and full disclosure are essential. Researchers must declare all potential conflicts to the relevant authorities, such as IRBs, and these declarations should be made public. Additionally, funding sources for research must be disclosed in all publications and presentations.

---

[9] https://code-medical-ethics.ama-assn.org/ethics-opinions/conflicts-interest-research (Accessed 1/28/24).
[10] Kondro, W. and Sibbald, B. (2004). Drug company experts advised staff to withhold data about SSRI use in children. *CMAJ*. 170(5):783. doi: 10.1503/cmaj.1040213. Erratum in: CMAJ. 2004 Apr 13; 170(8):1211.

The Importance of Continuing Education in Research Ethics

Continuing education in research ethics is crucial for physicians and researchers to stay abreast of evolving ethical standards and regulations. For instance, the emergence of new technologies like CRISPR gene editing poses novel ethical dilemmas. The case of Chinese scientist He Jiankui, who reportedly used CRISPR to genetically modify human embryos, resulted in widespread condemnation and highlighted the need for ongoing ethical education in emerging scientific fields.[11]

Regular training programs, workshops, and seminars on research ethics should be mandatory for all involved in medical research. These educational initiatives help reinforce the importance of ethical conduct and in understanding complex ethical issues in modern research.

Case Studies: Ethical Dilemmas and Resolutions in Recent Research

Case studies play a vital role in understanding and resolving ethical dilemmas in medical research. For example, the SUPPORT study (Surfactant, Positive Pressure, and Oxygenation Randomized Trial)[12] (seen in Chapter 10), which aimed to determine the optimal oxygen levels for premature infants, faced ethical scrutiny. The controversy centered around the adequacy of informed consent and the communication of risks to the

---

[11] Cyranoski, D. (2018). CRISPR-baby scientist fails to satisfy critics. *Nature*. 564. doi: 10.1038/d41586-018-07573-w.

[12] Stevens, T.P., Finer, N.N., Carlo, W.A., Szilagyi, P.G., Phelps, D.L., Walsh, M.C., Gantz, M.G., Laptook, A.R., Yoder, B.A., Faix, R.G., Newman, J.E., Das, A., Do, B.T., Schibler, K., Rich, W., Newman, N.S., Ehrenkranz, R.A., Peralta-Carcelen, M., Vohr, B.R., Wilson-Costello, D.E., Yolton, K., Heyne, R.J., Evans, P.W., Vaucher, Y.E., Adams-Chapman, I., McGowan, E.C., Bodnar, A., Pappas, A., Hintz, S.R., Acarregui, M.J., Fuller, J., Goldstein, R.F., Bauer, C.R., O'Shea, T.M., Myers, G.J. and Higgins, R.D. (Aug 2014). SUPPORT Study Group of the Eunice Kennedy Shriver National Institute of Child Health and Human Development Neonatal Research Network. Respiratory outcomes of the surfactant positive pressure and oximetry randomized trial (SUPPORT). *J Pediatr*. 165(2):240–249.e4. doi: 10.1016/j.jpeds.2014.02.054. Epub 2014 Apr 13.

parents. This case highlighted the complexities of informed consent in vulnerable populations and led to revisions in consent procedures.[13]

Another example is the Havasupai Tribe diabetes research case, where researchers used DNA samples provided for diabetes research to study schizophrenia and other genetic traits without the tribe's consent. This invasion of privacy, breach of trust, and consent led to a lawsuit and a settlement, underscoring the importance of clear and specific informed consent in research involving genetic material.[14]

These case studies demonstrate the ongoing challenges in ethical decision-making in medical research and the importance of learning from past mistakes to inform future practices.

Regulatory Frameworks and Institutional Oversight

The ethical conduct of medical research is underpinned by robust regulatory frameworks and institutional oversight mechanisms. These systems are designed to protect the rights and welfare of research participants and ensure the integrity of research practices.

IRBs are pivotal in safeguarding the rights and well-being of participants, acting as a check against potential ethical violations.

At the federal level, agencies like the U.S. Food and Drug Administration (FDA) provide guidelines and regulations for clinical trials, including requirements for testing new drugs and medical devices. The FDA's regulations are important for ensuring that medical products are both safe and effective before they become available to the public.

Internationally, organizations such as the World Health Organization (WHO) set standards and guidelines for health research. The WHO guidelines offer a global perspective on research ethics, addressing issues like equitable access to research benefits and the ethical conduct of research in

---

[13] Lantos, J.D. and Feudtner, C. (Jan–Feb 2015). SUPPORT and the ethics of study implementation: Lessons for comparative effectiveness research from the trial of oxygen therapy for premature babies. *Hastings Cent Rep.* 45(1):30–40. doi: 10.1002/hast.407. Epub 2014 Dec 19.

[14] Mello, M.M. and Wolf, L.E. (Jul 15 2010). The Havasupai Indian tribe case — lessons for research involving stored biologic samples. *N Engl J Med.* 363(3):204–207. doi: 10.1056/NEJMp1005203. Epub 2010 Jun 9.

low-resource settings. These international guidelines help harmonize ethical standards across different countries and cultural contexts.

Ethics committees in hospitals and research institutions serve as an additional layer of oversight. These committees, often comprising a diverse group of individuals including medical professionals, ethicists, and community representatives, provide guidance on ethical issues in patient care and research. They are instrumental in addressing complex ethical dilemmas, developing institutional policies, and providing education on ethical issues. In research, they complement the work of IRBs by focusing on broader ethical considerations and ensuring that the institution's research activities align with its ethical standards.

The regulatory frameworks and institutional oversight mechanisms, including IRBs, federal and international regulations, and ethics committees, form a comprehensive system for ensuring ethical conduct in medical research. They work collaboratively to protect research participants, uphold ethical standards, and maintain public trust in the medical research process.

Conclusion

Summarizing the importance of ethics in medical research

The exploration of ethical principles in medical research underscores their indispensable role in safeguarding the dignity, rights, and well-being of research participants. Ethics serve as the moral compass guiding researchers and physicians, ensuring that the pursuit of scientific knowledge is not at the expense of human values and welfare. The historical lessons, from the Tuskegee Syphilis Study to the DeepMind-NHS data privacy concerns, illustrate the potentially catastrophic consequences when ethical considerations are sidelined.

The ongoing need for vigilance and adaptation in ethical standards

Ethical vigilance in medical research is not a one-time effort but a continuous commitment. As medical science advances, bringing forth new technologies and methodologies, ethical standards must evolve to address emerging challenges. This includes adapting to innovations in genetics, AI, and globalized clinical trials, ensuring that ethical considerations keep pace with technological advancements. The role of regulatory bodies, IRBs, and ethics committees is imperative in this ongoing process, requiring constant reevaluation and updating of ethical guidelines.

Call to action for researchers and physicians

This chapter serves as a call to action for researchers and physicians to uphold and advocate for high ethical standards in medical research. It is a reminder of their dual responsibility to advance medical science while protecting the rights and interests of participants. Researchers and physicians must engage in continuous ethical education, remain vigilant against conflicts of interest, and actively participate in the ethical review process. They are the stewards of ethical research, and their commitment is vital in maintaining public trust and integrity in the field of medical science.

The ethical landscape of medical research is complex and ever-changing. It demands a concerted effort from all stakeholders in the medical community to ensure that research is conducted with the highest ethical standards, respecting the noble tradition of medicine and its primary goal — to benefit humanity.

Chapter 2

The Tuskegee Syphilis Study: A Legacy of Betrayal

Beneath the veneer of scientific inquiry and medical advancement, the Tuskegee Syphilis Study stands as a monument to the profound betrayal of trust and the egregious abuse of human rights. In the red earth of Alabama, shadows were cast not by the setting sun but by a decades-long experiment that saw African American men used as unwitting pawns in a cruel game of observation and neglect. Promised treatment for their afflictions, these men were instead left to the merciless progression of syphilis, their bodies and futures sacrificed at the altar of scientific curiosity. The horror of their ordeal, compounded by the stark injustice of their exploitation, is a reminder of the depths to which humanity can sink in the pursuit of knowledge. As we venture into the heart of this darkness, let us be guided by a resolve to confront the truths laid bare and a determination to ensure that such atrocities are never repeated.

The Tuskegee Syphilis Study, conducted from 1932 to 1972, is one of the most infamous chapters in the history of medical research, epitomizing a profound breach of ethical standards. Initiated and conducted by the U.S. Public Health Service (USPHS), the study involved tracking the natural progression of untreated syphilis in African American men in Tuskegee, Alabama, under the guise of providing free healthcare (see Figure 1).[1]

---

[1] Brandt, A.M. (December 1978). Racism and research: The case of the Tuskegee Syphilis study. *The Hastings Center Report*, 8(6):21–29.

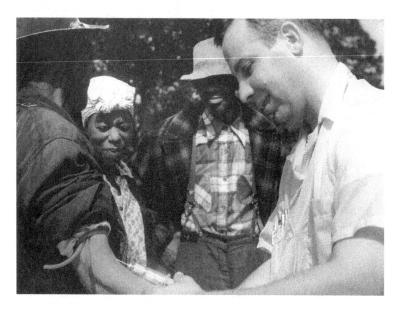

Figure 1.   A doctor drawing blood from a patient as part of the Tuskegee Syphilis Study.
Source: Image from the National Archives of Atlanta, GA, Public Domain.

The study enrolled African American men, nearly two-thirds of whom had syphilis. Public health workers went into the community to test patients for syphilis and enroll them in the study (Figure 1). These men were not told what disease they had, instead, they were told they were being treated for "bad blood," a local term used for various ailments. The researchers did not provide them with the proper treatment even after penicillin became the standard and effective treatment for syphilis in the 1940s. The study continued for 40 years, during which the participants were deprived of essential medical treatment, leading to severe health consequences, including death.[2]

The Tuskegee Syphilis Study was initiated at a time when syphilis was a major public health concern. In the early 20th century, syphilis was a widespread and serious disease for which there were limited treatments. The USPHS was particularly interested in understanding the progression of untreated syphilis. At that time, the long-term effects of the disease

---

[2]Reverby, S.M. (2009). *Examining Tuskegee: The Infamous Syphilis Study and Its Legacy.* The University of North Carolina Press.

were not well understood, and there was a significant interest in studying its natural history, especially since treatment options were limited and often ineffective.

Macon County, Alabama, was chosen for the Tuskegee Syphilis Study for several reasons. First, the county had a high prevalence of syphilis among its African American population. This high incidence rate provided a sufficient sample size for the study. Second, the socio-economic conditions and the existing racial inequalities in Macon County made it easier for the researchers to recruit and retain participants. Many of the men enrolled in the study were poor, had limited access to health-care, and were thus more likely to agree to participate in exchange for free medical exams, meals, and burial insurance, which were offered as incentives.

The choice of Macon County and the African American population for the study was also influenced by prevailing racial prejudices and ste-reotypes. At the time, there were misconceptions and biases about the susceptibility and response to syphilis in different races, which played a role in the selection of the study group.

At the time the study began, the scientific community's understanding of syphilis and its treatment was evolving. The Tuskegee Study was ini-tially designed to record the natural history of syphilis in hopes of justify-ing treatment programs for African Americans. However, as the study progressed, it became less about understanding the disease and more about observing the effects of untreated syphilis, without regard for the human cost.

The study took place in an era marked by racial discrimination, which played a significant role in the selection of the study subjects and their exploitation. The researchers took advantage of the participants' socio-economic status and the prevalent racial inequalities, betraying their trust and violating basic ethical principles of medicine and research.[3]

The Tuskegee Syphilis Study's legacy is now synonymous with ethi-cal violations in medical research and is a stark reminder of the impor-tance of ethical standards in medical research. It led to public outrage and significant changes in research ethics and regulations, including the

---

[3] Jones, J.H. (1981). *Bad Blood: The Tuskegee Syphilis Experiment*. The Free Press.

requirement for informed consent and the establishment of Institutional Review Boards (IRBs) to oversee research involving human subjects.[4]

The Tuskegee Syphilis Experiment, initiated in 1932 by the USPHS and led by Dr. Taliaferro Clark, was conceived to study the natural progression of untreated syphilis in African American men and the practicality of and effectiveness of mass control of syphilis. This study was based in Macon County, Alabama. Macon County was the poorest county in Alabama and had the highest prevalence rate of syphilis, approximately 40%. Macon County was also chosen because of its proximity to the Tuskegee Institute and its hospital, the John A. Andrew Hospital, and the Tuskegee Veterans Administration Hospital, which were both African-American-run institutions.

The USPHS aimed to document the full course of the disease, ostensibly to understand the need for treatment programs for African Americans. The researchers chose African American men as subjects, exploiting prevalent racial and socio-economic disparities. The recruitment of these men was based on deception. The USPHS capitalized on the lack of healthcare access in the African American community and misled the participants by offering what was presented as free healthcare from the government.

The study initially involved 600 black men: 399 with syphilis and 201 who were not infected. The study's design did not include informed consent. The infected men were not informed that they had syphilis, nor were they informed about the true nature of the study.

One of the most egregious aspects of the study was the denial of treatment to the participants. By 1947, penicillin had become the standard and effective treatment for syphilis. However, the men in the Tuskegee Study were not offered this treatment. The researchers went to great lengths to ensure that the participants did not receive penicillin, even intervening to prevent them from being drafted during World War II, as the military would have required a medical examination and likely treated any cases of syphilis (see footnote 2).

---

[4]White, R.M. (2005). *The Tuskegee Syphilis Study: The Real Story and Beyond. Montgomery.* NewSouth Books.

The researchers justified their deception by the scientific aim of the study, which was to observe the natural progression of untreated syphilis. This rationale was used to continue the study long after effective treatment was available, reflecting a severe breach of ethical standards in medical research (see footnote 1).

The USPHS researchers, instead of providing the necessary treatment, observed the men as the disease progressed, leading to severe health complications, including blindness, mental illness, and death (see footnote 2).

Several key figures were instrumental in the design and implementation of the Tuskegee Syphilis Experiment, each playing a distinct role in its execution.

Dr. Taliaferro Clark (Figure 2): As the originator of the study, Dr. Clark was a key figure in its inception. He was a Public Health Service officer who initially conceptualized the study. Clark's role was pivotal in the early stages of the experiment, particularly in establishing its framework and objectives. His involvement set the stage for a study that would become one of the most controversial in medical history.

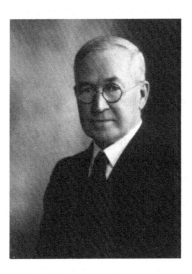

Figure 2.   Dr. Taliaferro Clark.

Source: The National Library of Medicine, public domain.

Dr. Taliaferro Clark's motivation for initiating the Tuskegee Syphilis Study was primarily scientific and public health-oriented. As a senior officer in the USPHS, Dr. Clark was interested in understanding the natural progression of untreated syphilis, particularly in African American populations.

At the time the study was conceived in the early 1930s, syphilis was a significant public health issue, and there was limited understanding of its progression and long-term effects, especially among African Americans. Dr. Clark and his colleagues at the USPHS saw an opportunity to study the disease's natural history in a population with a high incidence of syphilis.

The rationale was that by observing the untreated course of syphilis, they could gather valuable data that would inform future treatment strategies and public health interventions. This was deemed particularly important because effective treatments for syphilis were not yet available when the study began.

However, it is important to note that while the scientific intent might have been to advance medical understanding, the study was fundamentally flawed in its ethical design. The participants were not informed of their condition and were misled about the nature of the study, violating basic principles of informed consent and medical ethics. Dr. Clark's motivations, though rooted in public health concerns, led to one of the most notorious ethical breaches in medical research history. Dr. Clark died in 1948.

Dr. Oliver C. Wenger (Figure 3), a physician with the USPHS, played a significant role in the Tuskegee Syphilis Study, a role that has since been scrutinized for its ethical implications. Wenger, whose medical career was centered around public health and epidemiology, particularly in sexually transmitted infections, was deeply involved in the study's implementation and operational oversight.

In the Tuskegee Study, Wenger's responsibilities extended to crucial aspects such as participant recruitment and management. He was instrumental in selecting the African American men from Macon County, Alabama, and played a key role in designing the study's methodology. His operational oversight included coordinating with other staff, ensuring adherence to the study's protocols, and making pivotal decisions about its conduct.

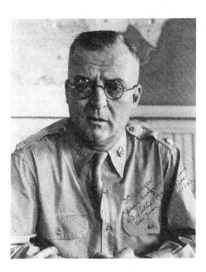

Figure 3. Oliver Wenger.
Source: Image from the National Library of Medicine, public domain.

One of the most significant and ethically questionable decisions made during the study, in which Wenger was involved, was the choice to continue the study without treating the infected participants with penicillin, once it became available as an effective treatment for syphilis. This decision, made for the sake of the study's objectives, represented a major ethical lapse and has been a focal point of criticism in subsequent analyses of the study.

Wenger's actions during the Tuskegee Syphilis Study, particularly considering the evolving ethical standards over the decades of the study, have contributed to the discourse on medical ethics and the responsibilities inherent in medical research. His involvement in the study is often cited in historical and ethical studies as an example of the complexities and ethical challenges in public health research.

Eunice Rivers (Figure 4), an African-American public health nurse and scientific assistant, was employed by the USPHS and was a key figure in the Tuskegee Study from its inception in 1932 until its end in 1972.

Starting in January 1923, Nurse Eunice Rivers began her work with the Tuskegee Institute Movable School. In this role, she delivered a range of public health services to African-American communities in rural Alabama. Her work with the school established her as a respected health authority

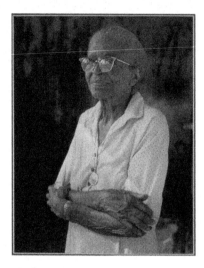

Figure 4.   Eunice Rivers.
Source: https://commons.wikimedia.org/wiki/Category:Eunice_Rivers_Laurie.

among African-American farming families in and around Tuskegee, Alabama, where she became a trusted figure in the community.[5]

Rivers was instrumental in recruiting the African American men who formed the study's participant group. Her status as a respected and trusted member of the local community in Macon County, Alabama, was leveraged to gain the trust of potential participants. She played a significant role in convincing these men to join the study, often under the impression that they would receive beneficial medical treatment for their "bad blood." During the Great Depression, African-Americans who could not afford healthcare joined Miss Rivers' Lodge (the study group) where they would obtain free physical exams at Tuskegee University along with hot meals and rides to and from the clinic.

Liaison Between Researchers and Participants

As the study progressed, Rivers became the primary liaison between the researchers and the participants. She was responsible for maintaining

---

[5] Smith, S.L. (1996). Neither victim nor villain: Nurse Eunice Rivers, the Tuskegee syphilis experiment, and public health work. *Journal of Women's History*, 8(1): 95–113. doi: 10.1353/jowh.2010.0446.

contact with the men, scheduling examinations, and ensuring their continued participation. Her familiarity with the community and her position as a healthcare provider helped in building and maintaining this crucial link.

Rivers' involvement in the Tuskegee Study raises complex ethical questions. On one hand, she was seen as a caregiver dedicated to her patients, and on the other, she was a key figure in a study that is now widely recognized as a significant ethical violation. Understanding her motivations is challenging. Some argue that Rivers, like many medical professionals of her time, may have believed in the scientific value of the study and trusted the judgment of the researchers. Others suggest that her actions were influenced by the hierarchical and racial dynamics of the time, which could have limited her autonomy and decision-making power.

After the study's unethical nature was publicly exposed in 1972, Rivers faced significant criticism. She was often portrayed as complicit in the study's ethical breaches. This scrutiny has led to a re-evaluation of her role, considering the broader context of her position as a black woman in a segregated society, working within a government institution during a time when racial and gender biases were prevalent.

Nurse Eunice Rivers' role in the Tuskegee Syphilis Study is a reminder of the complex interplay between individual actions and systemic factors in medical research. Her involvement highlights the importance of ethical training and awareness for all healthcare professionals, regardless of their role in the research process. Rivers' story is a crucial part of the Tuskegee Study's legacy, contributing to our understanding of the ethical responsibilities of healthcare providers in research settings.

These individuals, among others, were central to the Tuskegee Syphilis Study's design and implementation. Their roles highlight the complexities and ethical dilemmas faced by medical professionals when personal and professional ethics collide with the demands of scientific research.

The involvement of these key figures in the Tuskegee Syphilis Study has been a subject of extensive analysis and criticism, particularly in how their actions and decisions contributed to one of the most egregious breaches of ethical conduct in medical research.

The Tuskegee Syphilis Study, conducted by the USPHS, is a profound example of ethical misconduct and racial exploitation in medical research.

A fundamental ethical violation in the Tuskegee Study was the lack of informed consent. The participants were not informed that they had syphilis and were misled to believe they were receiving treatment for "bad blood." This deception directly contravened the principles of informed consent, which require that participants be fully informed about the nature of the study, including any risks and the true nature of their condition. The study's continuation without informed consent, even after the establishment of such principles in documents like the Nuremberg Code (1947), highlights a severe breach of ethical medical practice (see footnote 1).

The selection of African American men as subjects for the study was influenced by the racial prejudices of the time. The researchers exploited the socio-economic vulnerabilities and the limited access to healthcare of the African American community in Macon County. This choice reflects the broader societal racial inequalities and the misconception that the progression of diseases like syphilis could vary based on race. The study's design and execution are examples of how racial biases can lead to exploitation in medical research (see footnote 2).

The USPHS exploited the trust of the African American community in Macon County. Nurse Eunice Rivers, a trusted figure in the community, played a key role in recruiting and retaining participants, furthering this breach of trust. The USPHS's actions undermined the community's trust in the healthcare system, with long-lasting implications for public health engagement in African American communities (see footnotes 1 and 2).

The Tuskegee Syphilis Study had profound and lasting effects on the participants, their families, the broader African American community, and public trust in medical institutions.

The health consequences for the men involved in the Tuskegee Study were devastating. As they were not treated for syphilis, many suffered from severe health complications associated with the disease, including neurological and cardiovascular damage, blindness, and premature death. The impact extended to their families, with the potential for congenital syphilis affecting their children. The betrayal felt by the participants and their families contributed to a deep-seated mistrust of medical institutions (see footnotes 1 and 2).

The Tuskegee Study significantly contributed to lasting mistrust in the African American community toward medical institutions and public health initiatives. This mistrust is often cited as a factor in the reluctance of African Americans to participate in medical research or seek routine medical care, impacting public health outcomes in the community. The study became emblematic of racial exploitation in medical research and healthcare, reinforcing existing fears and suspicions about the healthcare system among African Americans.[6]

The public revelation of the Tuskegee Study in 1972 led to widespread outrage and a reevaluation of research ethics and regulations. This outcry was a catalyst for significant changes, including the passage of the National Research Act in 1974 and the establishment of the National Commission for the Protection of Human Subjects of Biomedical and Behavioral Research. These developments led to the creation of the Belmont Report in 1979,[7] which laid out fundamental ethical principles for conducting research involving human subjects, emphasizing informed consent, beneficence, and justice.

The Tuskegee Study egregiously violated fundamental ethical principles, including respect for persons, beneficence, and justice. The deception practiced on the study's participants, the denial of effective treatment, and the exploitation of a vulnerable population based on race represent a significant departure from the ethical conduct expected in medical research. This study is often cited as one of the most flagrant examples of ethical misconduct in the history of medical research, highlighting the dangers of valuing scientific inquiry over human dignity and welfare.

The Tuskegee Syphilis Study underscores the enduring need for vigilance in ethical conduct in medical research. It serves as a reminder that ethical considerations must be at the forefront of all medical research endeavors to prevent such tragedies from recurring. The study highlights the importance of continuous education, ethical training, and awareness among researchers and healthcare professionals. It also emphasizes the

---

[6]Gamble, V.N. (1997). Under the shadow of Tuskegee: African Americans and health care. *American Journal of Public Health*, 87(11):1773–1778.

[7]The Belmont Report (2014). Ethical principles and guidelines for the protection of human subjects of research. *The Journal of the American College of Dentists*, 81(3) (Summer): 4–13. PMID: 25951677 (Department of Health, Education, and Welfare; National Commission for the Protection of Human Subjects of Biomedical and Behavioral Research).

need for a robust system of checks and balances, including institutional review boards and ethical committees, to ensure that the rights and well-being of research participants are always protected.

The Tuskegee Syphilis Study is not just a historical case of ethical violation but a continuing call to action for the medical research community to uphold the highest standards of ethical conduct. It is a reminder that the pursuit of knowledge should never come at the cost of human rights and dignity.

Chapter 3

The Guatemala Syphilis Experiment: Cross-Border Ethical Violations

In a quiet corner of Guatemala, a story unfolded that would later shake the very foundations of medical ethics and human rights. Orchestrated by American researchers in the mid-20th century, the Guatemala Syphilis Experiment was a study that crossed lines many never knew existed. Here, without consent or knowledge, individuals became subjects in a harrowing investigation into syphilis, their bodies unknowingly enlisted in a battle against a disease with no intention of providing a cure. This chapter delves into the heart of this disturbing narrative, revealing the stark realities of exploitation under the guise of scientific progress. As you embark on this journey, be prepared to encounter a tale of profound ethical transgressions, one that challenges us to question the very essence of morality in the pursuit of knowledge.

The Guatemala Syphilis Experiment was carried out from 1946 to 1948. At the time, the US was worried about how to treat the GIs returning home with sexually transmitted diseases. To test the effectiveness of the new antibiotic, Penicillin, members of the US Public Health Service (USPHS) infected more than 1,300 Guatemalans with syphilis, gonorrhea, and chancroid.

The experiment was orchestrated primarily under the aegis of Dr. John Cutler, a USPHS physician. Cutler was a prestigious physician in his time. He received his medical degree from the Case Western Reserve University Medical School and joined the Public Health Service in 1942 where he

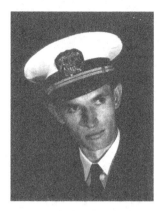

Figure 1.   Dr. John Cutler.
Source: Image from the National Library of Medicine, public Domain.

became interested in the treatment of sexually transmitted diseases. He eventually became Assistant Surgeon General of the United States.

Dr. Cutler (Figure 1), who later became infamously associated with the Tuskegee Syphilis Study, led the charge into a series of human experiments that would now be considered egregious violations of human rights and ethics.

The backdrop of these experiments was a post-World War II era, a time when the Nuremberg Code was in its nascency, and the world was grappling with the ethical breaches of the Nazi Regime. The fact that these experiments took place in the shadow of such a global moral reckoning further underscores the depth of their ethical transgressions.

Dr. Cutler was not new to this type of unacceptable research. In 1943 and 1944, he supervised experiments at the Terre Haute federal penitentiary, where inmates consented to be injected with gonorrhea strains. In exchange, they were promised $100, a certificate of merit, and a recommendation letter for the parole board. However, these experiments were halted when Cutler's superior concluded that the method used to induce gonorrhea in humans was unreliable, rendering the tests for prophylactic agents inconclusive.

Consequently, the research was transferred to Guatemala. Details of these experiments remained undisclosed to the public for over sixty years. Even now, there is limited awareness about these grave breaches of medical ethics and human rights.[1] The methods employed were not only unconsented but also underhanded, leveraging the vulnerability of marginalized populations. The researchers targeted those with diminished autonomy and societal power — individuals who were incapable of providing informed consent or who were coerced into participation through manipulation or outright deceit. The study encompassed over 5,128 individuals, including children, orphans, child and adult sex workers, Guatemalan Indigenous peoples, individuals with leprosy, psychiatric patients, inmates, and military personnel. In total, the experiments involved the intentional exposure of approximately 1308 individuals to syphilis, with a larger group subjected to diagnostic testing without their informed consent.[2] Included in this study were orphans as young as 9 years old.[3] One of the victims, Marta Orellana, recalled to a reporter that when she was a young girl living in an orphanage, she was summoned to the infirmary. She was brought into a room with two white men she had never met before and was instructed to lie down and open her legs. When she refused, she was slapped and was forced to comply with a procedure that infected her with syphilis (see footnote 3). She was never told who the men were or what they were doing to her.

In this study, after an infection was established, the patients were supposed to be treated with penicillin to eradicate the infection. However, not all patients were treated. Of the 1,308 people who were infected with a sexually transmitted disease, only 678 individuals were documented as receiving some form of treatment.[4] Some individuals, such as a patient known only as Berta, did not receive treatment until three months after her initial infection, and even then, the treatment came too late to prevent

---

[1] Reverby, S.M. (2011) "Normal exposure" and inoculation syphilis: APHS "Tuskegee" doctor in Guatemala, 1946–1948. *J Policy History*, 23(1):6–28.

[2] McGreal, C. (October 1, 2010). US says sorry for 'outrageous and abhorrent' Guatemalan syphilis tests. *The Guardian*.

[3] Rory, C. (8 June 2011) Guatemala victims of US syphilis study still haunted by the "devil's experiment", *The Guardian*.

[4] This is according to contemporaneous Cutler notes. PCSBI. (2011). Subject Database. chrome-extension://efaidnbmnnnibpcajpcglclefindmkaj/https://bioethicsarchive.george town.edu/pcsbi/sites/default/files/Ethically%20Impossible%20(with%20linked%20histori cal%20documents)%202.7.13.pdf (Accessed 6/14/24).

severe medical consequences and her subsequent death. Furthermore, the overall approach of the researchers was to intentionally infect participants and, as a general practice, leave them untreated to observe the progress of the disease, which was an explicit deviation from ethical medical standards and human rights.

The choice of populations — prisoners, psychiatric patients, soldiers, and sex workers — was not incidental but a calculated decision that preyed upon individuals less likely to have access to legal or social recourse. It reflected an underlying utilitarian philosophy that deemed certain lives less valuable, a viewpoint sharply inimical to the foundational medical ethic of "do no harm", but very much in the Nazi worldview of *Lebensunwertes leben*, or "life unworthy of life."[5] The individuals were chosen not only for their perceived disposability but also for logistical convenience, as they could be monitored and controlled within institutional settings. This deliberate targeting of powerless groups starkly violates the principle of justice, which requires fair treatment and respect for everyone, regardless of their social standing or personal situations. When picturing the Guatemala experiments, it's important not to confuse them with the polished, well-equipped labs often seen in Hollywood depictions of medical research. Far from being conducted in bright, sterile rooms with doctors in white coats, these experiments took place in prison cells, orphanages, and rural clinics. The methods used were far from the standard medical practices like pinprick vaccinations or oral medication. Instead, the researchers employed harmful techniques to administer STD-causing bacteria, targeting individuals who were already in distressing situations. This approach not only disregarded their well-being but also exacerbated their existing suffering. This can be seen in this excerpt from the president's report on these experiments.

"Berta was a female patient in the psychiatric hospital. Her age and the illness that brought her to the hospital are unknown. In February 1948, Berta was injected in her left arm with syphilis. A month later, she developed scabies (an itchy skin infection caused by a mite). Several weeks later, (lead investigator Dr. John) Cutler noted that she had also developed

---

[5] Kater, M.H. (2000). *Doctors Under Hitler.* Chapel Hill, NC. The University of North Carolina Press.

red bumps where he had injected her arm, lesions on her arms and legs, and her skin was beginning to waste away from her body. Berta was not treated for syphilis until three months after her injection. Soon after, on August 23, Dr. Cutler wrote that Berta appeared as if she was going to die, but he did not specify why, nor did he suggest that she be evaluated or receive treatment. However, that same day he put gonorrheal pus from another male subject into both of Berta's eyes, as well as in her urethra and rectum. He also reinfected her with syphilis. Several days later, Berta's eyes were filled with pus from the gonorrhea, and she was bleeding from her urethra. On August 27, Berta died."[6]

Getting more information about the other patients in these studies is difficult as detailed public records on the health outcomes or post-study care of individual victims are scarce. The privacy of medical records and the passage of time make it challenging to trace the long-term health impacts on the study's subjects and their communities.

In the shadow of these experiments lies a somber lesson: the critical importance of ethical standards in medical research. The Guatemala Syphilis Experiment is a striking reminder of the potential for medical science to deviate into the realms of inhumanity when ethical considerations are cast aside. This chapter seeks to expose this dark chapter of medical history, not only to bear witness to the wrongs of the past but also to illuminate the path toward a more ethical and humane practice of medicine.

The Guatemala Syphilis Experiment was not just a mere footnote in medical history but a profound example of ethical transgression. The experimental procedures were a harrowing breach of medical ethics and human rights. Dr. John Cutler, the principal investigator, employed various inoculation methods, including direct exposure of subjects to syphilis. Prostitutes, who were also intentionally infected, were used to transfer the disease to subjects such as prisoners and psychiatric patients, without their knowledge or consent (see footnote 2).

In a methodical and chillingly clinical manner, treatments were administered only to a subset of those infected, ostensibly to test the efficacy of penicillin. However, records suggest that many subjects received

---

[6] Ethically Impossible STD Research in Guatemala from 1946–1948. Presidential commission for the Study of Bioethical Issues (see footnote 4).

no treatment whatsoever, turning them into mere data points in a medical study utterly devoid of compassion or ethical consideration. The Tuskegee Syphilis Study, conducted contemporaneously in the United States, presents a disturbing parallel. In Tuskegee, African American men with existing syphilis infections were observed without being offered effective treatment, under the guise of studying the natural progression of the disease. While both studies operated under a veil of scientific inquiry, they shared a common thread of exploiting weak and unprotected populations — a violation distinctly at odds with the ethical principle of justice, which demands equal respect and treatment for all individuals.

The contrasts between the two are equally telling. The Tuskegee Experiment withheld treatment to study disease progression, while in Guatemala, the syphilis bacteria were deliberately introduced to subjects. Both studies, however, were unified by their fundamental breach of informed consent, a cornerstone of ethical medical practice.

The Guatemala Syphilis Experiment underscores an obligation for current and future healthcare professionals: to steadfastly uphold ethical principles and advocate for the rights and dignity of all patients. This historical episode stands as an enduring lesson that the end never justifies the means in medical practice, and it is through the lens of these ethical principles that such atrocities must be examined and remembered.

As was stated in the 2011 Presidential Commission for the Study of Bioethical Issues (see footnote 4), sound scientific experimentation inherently involves uncertainty, and it's impossible to completely shield volunteers from all physical or psychological risks. However, for research involving human subjects to be ethical, several key principles must be adhered to. First, participants must be volunteers who have given their informed consent. They should be treated with fairness and respect. The risks they are subjected to should be reasonable and balanced against the potential humanitarian benefits. Importantly, participants should not be used merely as a means to an end. In the absence of these ethical constraints, tragic results may follow.

The Guatemala Syphilis Experiment represents a monumental failure of ethical constraint, particularly concerning the autonomy and dignity of individuals. Consent procedures were not just inadequately followed; they were entirely disregarded. Informed consent, the process by which patients are educated about the risks, benefits, and alternatives to a proposed treatment or intervention, is fundamental to ethical medical practice. This fundamental principle was bypassed entirely in the Guatemala experiments, as subjects were neither informed of the nature and risks of the experiments nor allowed to agree or decline participation (see footnote 4).

The ethical implications of such actions are profound. By depriving individuals of the right to make informed decisions about their own bodies, the researchers treated them as means to an end, violating their basic human rights and the ethical principle of respect for persons. This lapse not only undermines the trust between healthcare providers and patients but also compromises the integrity of the medical profession itself.

The exploitation of vulnerable populations — specifically the mentally ill and incarcerated — raises serious ethical concerns. These groups were specifically targeted due to their diminished autonomy and the convenience of their institutionalization. The mentally ill and incarcerated individuals often have limited capacity or freedom to provide informed consent, making them a population in need of greater protection rather than exploitation. This targeting breaches the principle of justice, mandating fair treatment for all individuals and extra safeguards for the most at risk. The Guatemala experiments exploited their vulnerability for convenience and because of the researchers' assumption that they would have less societal support or recourse, which compounds the ethical violation.[7]

Healthcare professionals must always advocate for the rights of their patients, ensuring that they are treated with respect and that their autonomy is honored. The lessons from the Guatemala Syphilis Experiment must not be forgotten. They serve as a powerful reminder of the critical importance of informed consent and the protection of defenseless populations in medical research and practice.

The Tuskegee Experiment only became well known after a report by the journalist Jean Heller of the Associated Press. In 1972, she revealed that the subjects of the Tuskegee program went untreated. In

---

[7]Michael A.R. MD, MPH, and Robert G. JD. (2013). First, do no harm: The US sexually transmitted disease experiments in Guatemala. *Am J Public Health,*103:2122–2126. doi: 10.2105/AJPH.2013.301520.

comparison, the Guatemala Experiment went unremarked for 60 years. In 2010, Professor Susan M. Reverby, a historian at Wellesley College, published a report on the topic. During her research on the Tuskegee Experiment, Reverby came across archived documents belonging to Dr. Cutler. These documents detailed the unethical practices used in the Guatemalan study.

The Guatemala Syphilis Experiment was kept secret for decades, avoiding public scrutiny. However, once details emerged, the response was one of widespread condemnation. Upon exposure of the nature of the Guatemala experiments, there was a universal outcry from the media, which played a crucial role in bringing the issue to light, generating public discourse, and demanding accountability. The scientific community, shaken by the revelations, was prompted to reassess ethical standards.

The Guatemala Syphilis Experiment's ethical breaches significantly influenced revisions to the Declaration of Helsinki, a cornerstone of international research ethics. The World Medical Association recognizing the importance of transparency created provisions in the Helsinki Declaration for the public registration of research and the publication of results, including negative and inconclusive findings. This openness is intended to promote accountability, allow for public scrutiny, and ensure that the research contributes to the broader body of scientific knowledge.

Further, the experiment's violation of informed consent principles led to stricter guidelines ensuring consent is voluntary, informed, and can be withdrawn at any time. It also highlighted the need for special protections for vulnerable populations, ensuring research involving them is directly beneficial and conducted with extra care. In response to the experiment's lack of ethical oversight, the declaration now mandates that all human research be reviewed and approved by an independent committee before it begins, such as institutional review boards (IRBs) or ethics committees, to ensure that ethical standards are upheld.[8]

Lastly, the neglect of post-study care for participants in Guatemala has been addressed by stipulating researchers' obligations to provide access to effective interventions post-research, ensuring participants are

---

[8] https://www.wma.net/what-we-do/medical-ethics/declaration-of-helsinki/doh-oct2008/ (Accessed 6/14/24).

not left worse off. These revisions to the Declaration of Helsinki reflect a global commitment to learning from past mistakes and safeguarding the dignity, rights, and welfare of research participants.

The Guatemala Syphilis Experiment stands as a graphic violation of the four fundamental principles of biomedical ethics: autonomy, beneficence, non-maleficence, and justice.

- **Autonomy:** This principle emphasizes the right of individuals to make informed decisions about their own healthcare. In the Guatemala experiments, this principle was violated as subjects were not informed about the nature of the experiments nor were they given the opportunity to consent or refuse participation.
- **Beneficence:** Healthcare providers are obligated to act in the best interest of the patient, providing benefits while balancing risks. The experiments' designers ostensibly aimed to understand and improve treatment for STDs, but they did so at the expense of their subjects' well-being, thereby contravening this principle.
- **Non-maleficence:** The directive to "do no harm" is a foundational medical ethic. The deliberate infection of individuals with syphilis and other STDs without their consent constitutes a direct breach of this ethical tenet.
- **Justice:** This principle demands fair and equitable treatment of all individuals. The targeting of vulnerable populations in the experiments, such as prisoners and psychiatric patients, represents a profound injustice, as these groups were selected due to their diminished ability to resist or advocate for themselves.

Today's ethical standards, influenced by documents such as the Declaration of Helsinki and the Belmont Report, would unequivocally condemn the Guatemala Syphilis Experiment. Contemporary ethics demands rigorous informed consent processes, unbiased selection of research subjects, and IRB oversight to ensure the rights and welfare of participants are protected.

Modern ethical scrutiny would also consider the broader social implications of research, including the potential for stigmatization and long-term societal impacts. In the current ethical climate, an experiment of the nature of the Guatemala Syphilis Experiment would not only be deemed unethical but also likely be illegal, facing universal condemnation and legal repercussions.

The Guatemala Syphilis Experiment serves as a reminder of the critical importance of ethical oversight in research and the ongoing need to prioritize the rights and dignity of all individuals in medical practice. As healthcare professionals and researchers, it is imperative to internalize the lessons of the past to guide future conduct, ensuring that all medical interventions adhere to the highest ethical standards.

The USPHS played a central role in the Guatemala Syphilis Experiment, with its involvement rooted in the era's public health agenda. At the time, the USPHS was actively seeking methods to control the spread of sexually transmitted diseases, which were considered a significant threat to public health and military efficiency. Dr. John Cutler, an employee of the USPHS, was the leading figure of the experiment and was acting under the direction and endorsement of this government institution.

The USPHS's responsibility in this unethical experimentation is twofold. First, it provided the structure and resources that enabled the experimentation. Second, it failed to enforce the necessary ethical oversight to prevent such abuses from occurring. The institution's direct involvement and the subsequent lack of appropriate response reflect a systemic failure to protect individuals' rights and welfare.

Scientific research demands considerable investment from society, often competing with other valuable activities that contribute to public welfare. Consequently, the public is entitled to transparency and accountability regarding how resources dedicated to scientific pursuits are utilized and managed, especially when these pursuits aim to benefit the common good. This need for accountability becomes even more critical in cases where publicly funded research involves human participants.

The USPHS was not the only institution responsible for the abuses in this experiment (see Figure 2). Several other US, Guatemalan, and international organizations share the blame. These include the Pan American Sanitary Bureau, the Guatemalan Government, and the National Institutes of Health (NIH).

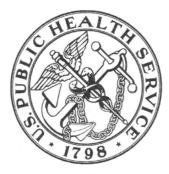

Figure 2. The seal of the US Public Health Service.
Source: Wikimedia Commons.

The Pan American Sanitary Bureau, which is now known as the Pan American Health Organization (PAHO), played a significant role in the Guatemala Syphilis Experiment during the late 1940s. As the regional office for the Americas of the World Health Organization (WHO), its involvement in facilitating these experiments underscores the complexity of international collaboration in public health initiatives, especially those involving human subjects.

The Bureau's support for the experiments was multifaceted, encompassing logistical assistance, provision of resources, and possibly the endorsement that lent the experiments an air of legitimacy within the international public health community. This support was crucial in establishing the groundwork for the experiments, enabling researchers, including Dr. John Cutler, to carry out their work under the guise of advancing medical knowledge and public health.

One of the ways the Pan American Sanitary Bureau contributed to the execution of the study was through its connections with local health authorities in Guatemala. These relationships were instrumental in gaining access to the populations that were subjected to the experiments, including prisoners, psychiatric patients, and soldiers. The Bureau's involvement likely facilitated negotiations with Guatemalan officials and institutions, ensuring that the research team had the necessary permissions and access to carry out their activities.

Moreover, the Bureau's role in the experiments reflects the broader issues of ethical oversight and accountability in international health research. At the time, the standards for informed consent and protection of human subjects were not as developed or universally enforced as they are today. The participation of a respected international organization in the experiments may have contributed to the oversight of ethical considerations, underlining the importance of robust ethical guidelines and accountability mechanisms in all forms of medical research.

The Guatemalan government and local health institutions played a pivotal role in the ethical breaches of the Guatemala Syphilis Experiment by allowing it on their soil and providing access to groups like prisoners, psychiatric patients, and soldiers without proper protection or informed consent. Their involvement highlights a significant lapse in ethical oversight and the protection of human rights, as they facilitated the USPHS researchers' access to state-run facilities and failed to safeguard their citizens against exploitation in medical research.

This complicity raises critical concerns about the responsibilities of host countries in international research collaborations, especially in protecting populations from unethical medical practices. The aftermath has underscored the urgent need for stronger ethical guidelines and oversight mechanisms globally to ensure the dignity and rights of research subjects are respected, reflecting on the complex dynamics of international research and the paramount importance of ethical conduct in medical studies.

The NIH is indirectly responsible for the abuses in the Guatemala Syphilis Experiment. Although there's no explicit documentation of the NIH's direct involvement in planning the experiments, its role in funding and overseeing research at the time implicates it in the broader failures of ethical oversight associated with the USPHS's activities.

The accountability measures for the Guatemala Syphilis Experiment have been subject to scrutiny and criticism. Many have argued that the US president's apology,[9] while necessary, is not sufficient as a sole measure of accountability. Victims and their families have sought legal redress and

---

[9] https://www.reuters.com/article/idUSTRE6903RZ/#:~:text=We%20deeply%20regret%20that%20it,case%20to%20an%20international%20court (Accessed 2/5/24).

compensation. In 2011, a lawsuit was filed against the U.S. government by victims and their families seeking compensation for the harm caused. However, a U.S. court dismissed the lawsuit, citing sovereign immunity, which protects the government from lawsuits without its consent.[10] Efforts to seek justice and compensation for the victims have continued, including calls for direct compensation and support for affected communities.

The USPHS, and by extension the U.S. government, faced a moral imperative to implement systemic changes in the wake of these revelations. This includes establishing and enforcing rigorous ethical guidelines, enhancing transparency in medical research, and ensuring that all research involving human subjects is subject to IRB review and follows the principles of informed consent, beneficence, non-maleficence, and justice. These changes were seen in the Belmont Report[11] and the report by the Presidential Commission for the Study of Bioethical Issues in 2011.[12]

The Guatemala Syphilis Experiment, a regrettable episode in medical history, teaches us crucial lessons while raising important questions for future research, particularly regarding ethical practices in contemporary medicine.

The experiment's blatant disregard for informed consent has reinforced its fundamental importance in medical research. It also highlighted the necessity for additional safeguards to protect susceptible groups, such as children, prisoners, and the mentally ill. This case demonstrated the critical need for stringent ethical oversight in research, leading to the strengthening of review boards and ethical committees to ensure that research protocols respect human dignity and rights. Furthermore, the international nature of this experiment prompted a reevaluation of global ethical standards in medical research, emphasizing the need for universally accepted ethical principles. The delayed revelation of the

---

[10] https://www.cnn.com/2012/01/10/world/americas/us-guatemala-std-experiments/index.html (Accessed 2/5/24).

[11] The Belmont Report (1979). National Commission for the Protection of Human Subjects of Biomedical and Behavioral Research. Ethical Principles and Guidelines for the Protection of Human Subjects of Research. U.S. Government Printing Office.

[12] Presidential Commission for the Study of Bioethical Issues. (2011). *"Ethically Impossible" STD Research in Guatemala from 1946 to 1948.*

experiment's details underscored the importance of transparency in research activities and accountability for ethical breaches.

However, this episode leaves us with several unanswered questions and areas for further exploration. The long-term psychological and physical impacts on the experiment's subjects remain unclear, raising questions about managing the aftermath of unethical research. The issue of institutional accountability for past unethical practices and measures to prevent future violations is another area needing attention. Additionally, incorporating cultural sensitivity and respect for local norms in international research settings is a growing concern. As medical technology and methodologies evolve, ethical standards must adapt to address new challenges. Finally, there is a need for educational initiatives in medical and research communities to prevent the recurrence of such ethical violations.

The existing system in the United States offers significant legal and regulatory safeguards for the health, rights, and welfare of individuals participating in research. Generally, this system functions to shield volunteers from harm or unethical treatment when they partake in scientific studies funded by the federal government.

In summary, while the Guatemala Syphilis Experiment serves as a clear reminder of the potential for atrocities in the absence of ethical vigilance, it also provides a platform for ongoing dialogue and improvement in medical research ethics. The lessons learned continue to shape our ethical frameworks, but the journey toward fully ethical research practices is an ongoing and necessary pursuit.

Chapter 4

The Willowbrook Experiments: Exploiting the Vulnerable

"Suffer the little children unto me."

Mark 10:14. KJV

Beneath the seemingly tranquil veneer of Willowbrook State School, a storm of ethical controversy brewed, one that would forever alter the landscape of medical research ethics. In the heart of this institution, a series of experiments unfolded that blurred the lines between medical advancement and moral transgression. The Willowbrook Hepatitis Experiments, conducted under the guise of scientific inquiry, subjected vulnerable residents to deliberate infection with hepatitis, sparking a nationwide debate on the rights of research subjects and the boundaries of ethical science. This chapter delves into the heart of Willowbrook's corridors, unraveling a narrative that is as compelling as it is disconcerting. Prepare to be drawn into a story that not only chronicles the pursuit of knowledge at a great and questionable cost but also serves as a pivotal lesson in the importance of safeguarding human dignity in the face of scientific exploration.

Willowbrook State School, often referred to as Willowbrook Hospital, was a state-supported institution for children with intellectual disabilities located in Staten Island, New York (Figure 1). It was the largest facility of its type in the world.

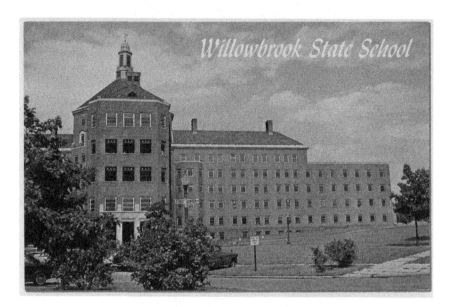

Figure 1. Willowbrook State School.
Source: Public domain — from The New York Public Library.

During the period between 1956 and 1971, Willowbrook became infamous not only for the controversial hepatitis experiments conducted on its residents but also for the deplorable conditions under which the children lived and were cared for.[1]
The facilities at Willowbrook were grossly inadequate and overcrowded. Originally designed to house fewer than its maximum capacity, by the early 1960s, it was home to over 6,200 residents, more than double its intended capacity. This severe overcrowding led to unsanitary conditions, with reports of children living in rooms smeared with feces and urine. The buildings were in a state of disrepair, with broken equipment and inadequate heating, contributing to an environment that was both physically unsafe and psychologically harmful. In an interview after an unplanned visit to the institution, Robert F. Kennedy (Figure 2), then a senator for the State of New York, referred to it as a "snake pit" and added that the children

---

[1] (January–February 1986). *Reviews of Infectious Diseases*. The University of Chicago. 8(1). All rights reserved. 0162-0886/86/0801-0015$02.00.

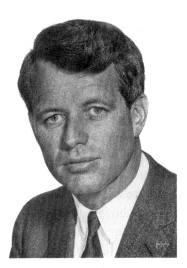

Figure 2. Robert F. Kennedy.
Source: Image from Wikicommons.

were "living in filth and dirt, their clothing in rags, in rooms less comfortable and cheerful than the cages in which we put animals in a zoo."[2]

The staffing levels at Willowbrook were critically low, often with one staff person to 40 residents. This staff-to-patient ratio made it impossible to maintain a clean and safe environment, much less offer individualized care or educational programming that was promised. There were not enough caregivers to attend to the basic needs of the children, let alone provide them with educational services, adequate medical care, or emotional support. Many of the staff were not trained to work with individuals with intellectual disabilities, further exacerbating the problems of neglect and mistreatment. This also contributed to the neglect and abuse of residents.

The care provided by the staff at Willowbrook was substandard, primarily due to the overwhelming number of residents and the lack of qualified personnel. Reports from the period describe a lack of basic hygiene care, with children often left in soiled clothing for extended periods. The

---

[2] https://www.nyc.gov/site/mopd/events/our-history.page?slide=10#:~:text=Robert%20
Kennedy%20toured%20the%20institution,put%20animals%20in%20a%20zoo.%22
(Accessed 2/20/24).

institution was also criticized for its use of physical restraints and sedation as a means of controlling behavior rather than addressing the underlying needs of the residents.[3] The nutritional and medical needs of the children were frequently neglected, leading to widespread illness and, in some cases, death.

The buildings at Willowbrook were not open to the public and were rarely visited by the facility's administration. William Bronston, a physician working there between 1968 and 1975, described the facility as "sealed off" and "living coffins for devalued people."[4] Dr. Bronson had toured facilities in Sweden where patients were treated with respect and educated to reach their potential. His goal was to bring reform to Willowbrook. When working within the system did not bring the results he had hoped for, he had his former teacher, Dr. Richard Koch, and a reporter for the Staten Island Advance, Jane Kurtin, visit Willowbrook. Kurtin's article, titled *Inside the Cages*, ran on the front page of the *Advance*. As a result, some parents began to complain about the conditions in the institution.

The conditions at Willowbrook State School were brought to public attention in 1972 by Geraldo Rivera, a journalist who investigated and produced a television expose titled "Willowbrook: The Last Great Disgrace."[5] His report, which included shocking footage of the overcrowded and unsanitary conditions, as well as the neglectful treatment of residents, sparked outrage and led to significant reforms in the care of people with intellectual disabilities.

Children placed in Willowbrook State School during the 1960s and 1970s were primarily individuals with intellectual and developmental disabilities. These children, ranging from infants to young adults, were placed in the institution for various reasons. The families place them there because of a lack of resources, support, or understanding in society.[6] The population at Willowbrook included children with a wide spectrum of

---

[3] https://www.nytimes.com/2020/02/21/nyregion/willowbrook-state-school-staten-island.html.

[4] The Path Forward. Remembering Willowbrook, https://www.youtube.com/watch?v=ev80q Etp2u4 (Accessed 1/31/24).

[5] Willowbrook:The Last Great Disgrace - Geraldo Rivera Documentary (1972). By Geraldo Rivera, WABC-TV Channel 7.

[6] https://disabilityjustice.org/the-closing-of-willowbrook/ (Accessed 2/2/24).

cognitive and physical disabilities, from mild learning disabilities to severe intellectual impairments, as well as those with conditions, such as Down syndrome, cerebral palsy, and autism.

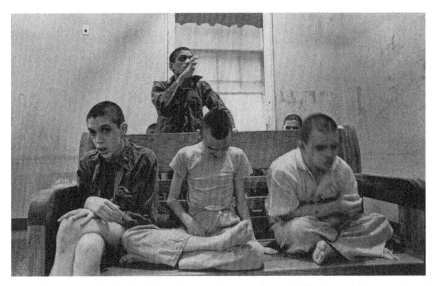

Photo from the College Of Staten Island's collection of Eric Aerts photographs of Willowbrook State School.
Source: Photo by Eric Aerts/Courtesy of Ericson Aerts and the College of Staten Island Archives & Special Collections.

Many families were advised by medical professionals or social workers to place their children in Willowbrook, being told it was the best option for their care and education. At the time, societal attitudes toward intellectual disabilities were less informed and supportive than they are today, and many families faced significant stigma and little assistance in caring for their disabled members. The promise of specialized care and schooling at Willowbrook was a compelling reason for many parents, who hoped for a better quality of life for their children.

However, once admitted to Willowbrook, the children often faced conditions that were far from the nurturing and therapeutic environment promised. Overcrowding, inadequate care, and neglect were rampant, exacerbated by the institution's insufficient resources and lack of qualified

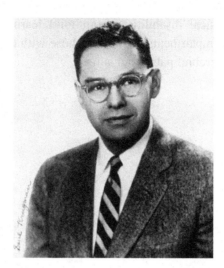

Figure 3.   Dr. Saul Krugman.

staff. The environment was not conducive to the development or well-being of the children, with many experiencing physical and psychological harm due to the conditions and treatment they endured.[7]

The children at Willowbrook were not just residents; they became subjects of medical experiments, most notably the hepatitis studies, without their or their guardians' informed consent. This further highlights the vulnerability and exploitation they faced, not only from the institution's living conditions but also from the very professionals entrusted with their care.

The Willowbrook hepatitis experiments were conducted from the 1950s through the early 1970s. They were led by Dr. Saul Krugman (Figure 3) and his team,[8] who aimed to understand the transmission of hepatitis, and its natural history, and to develop preventive measures, such as the use of gamma globulin. It was hoped that these studies would lead

---

[7] Rothman, D.J. and Rothman, S.M. (1984). *The Willowbrook Wars: Bringing the Mentally Disabled into the Community.* Harper & Row.

[8] Krugman, S., Giles, J.P. and Hammond, J. (1967). Infectious hepatitis: Evidence for two distinctive clinical, epidemiological, and immunological types of infection. *Journal of the American Medical Association*, 200(5):365–373.

to a vaccine against the disease. At the time, hepatitis was a significant health issue within institutions like Willowbrook, where outbreaks were common due to overcrowded and unsanitary conditions.

Saul Krugman's hepatitis experiments at Willowbrook State School were conducted in the context of research aimed at understanding and controlling hepatitis outbreaks within the institution.

These studies were not sponsored by a single entity but received support from various sources over time. Key sponsors and supporters of the research included the U.S. Army, the National Institutes of Health (NIH), and other public health entities interested in hepatitis research and vaccine development.

The U.S. Army's interest was partly due to the potential impact of hepatitis on military personnel, while the NIH, a major funding body for medical research in the United States, supported studies that promised to advance knowledge of infectious diseases and improve public health outcomes.[9]

In the Willowbrook experiments, the methods of exposing children to hepatitis varied. Some children were deliberately infected with the virus without receiving any globulin injections, which could potentially offer protection. Others received gamma globulin injections before being exposed to the virus. Additionally, some children were given the injections but were not exposed to the virus at all.[10] Each group was closely monitored by the medical team.

Children were infected with the hepatitis virus through several methods. In some cases, the virus was introduced through injections. In other cases, a particularly disturbing method of exposure was used, where the feces of residents already infected with hepatitis was mixed into chocolate milk, which was then given to the children participating in the study,

[9] Mays, J.B. and Hopper, K. (1996). The Agony of Willowbrook. In *Public Health Policies and Social Inequality*. New York. Cambridge University Press.

[10] Ward, R., Krugman, S., Giles, J.P., Jacobs, A.M. and Bodansky, O. (1958). Infectious hepatitis; Studies of its natural history and prevention. *N Engl J Med*. 258(9):407–416. doi: 10.1056/NEJM195802272580901.

without their knowledge of the contamination.[11,12] These methods of infection were based on the premise that exposing the children to the virus under controlled conditions would allow the researchers to observe the course of the disease and the body's immune response.

After being infected, the children were monitored for symptoms of hepatitis, and their medical conditions were documented by the research team. Those who developed the disease were observed to study the natural progression of hepatitis. The treatment provided to the children who became ill because of the experiments varied. While some received supportive care, the primary focus was on observing the natural course of the illness rather than actively treating the infection. The use of gamma globulin was part of the experiment to assess its effectiveness in preventing or ameliorating the disease, but it was not administered to all infected children.

In the context of the Willowbrook experiments, understanding the nature of hepatitis A and B is crucial. Hepatitis A, typically a self-limiting disease, presents with symptoms like fever, fatigue, and jaundice, and is more severe in adults than in children. Its mortality rate is low, with serious complications like fulminant hepatitis being rare. Hepatitis B, on the other hand, ranges from acute to chronic infections. Chronic hepatitis B can lead to serious conditions, such as cirrhosis, liver cancer, and liver failure. It's particularly dangerous when contracted at a young age, with a higher risk of chronic infection and associated mortality. In 2019, hepatitis B was responsible for approximately 820,000 deaths globally, primarily due to liver-related complications. This background is essential for understanding the implications and outcomes of the hepatitis studies conducted at Willowbrook State School.

---

[11] Rothman, D.J. (1982). Were Tuskegee & Willowbrook 'studies in nature'? *Hastings Cent Rep.* 12(2):5–7. PMID: 7096065.

[12] Rosenbaum, L. The Hideous Truths of Testing Vaccines on Humans, https://www.forbes.com/sites/leahrosenbaum/2020/06/12/willowbrook-scandal-hepatitis-experiments-hideous-truths-of-testing-vaccines-on-humans/?sh=443e6d4279c8 (Accessed 2/2/24).

The Researchers

Like many of the researchers profiled in this book, Drs. Krugman and Giles were intelligent and ambitious people, interested in advancing medicine and their careers. Like the others in this book, they were inured to the suffering of their patients and blind to their own ethical lapses.

Dr. Saul Krugman (1911–1995) was a pioneering American pediatrician and infectious disease specialist whose work significantly advanced the understanding and prevention of viral hepatitis.[13] Born in New York City, Krugman received his medical degree from New York University (NYU) School of Medicine in 1939. He served in the U.S. Army Medical Corps during World War II, where he first became interested in infectious diseases.

After the war, Krugman returned to NYU and Bellevue Hospital, where he began his research into infectious diseases, particularly focusing on hepatitis. His involvement in the Willowbrook hepatitis experiments during the 1950s and 1960s was controversial but led to critical discoveries about the transmission and prevention of hepatitis A and B. Krugman's work was instrumental in differentiating between these two types of hepatitis and in the development of the hepatitis B vaccine, a breakthrough that has saved countless lives worldwide.

Despite the ethical controversies surrounding his research methods, Krugman's contributions to medicine were recognized with numerous awards and honors, including the Albert Lasker Clinical Medical Research Award in 1972. (The Lasker Award is sometimes referred to as the Nobel Prize of Medicine.) He served as the president of the American Pediatric Society and was a member of various prestigious medical boards and committees. Krugman's legacy is marked by his significant contributions to the field of infectious diseases, albeit intertwined with ongoing debates about the ethics of his research practices.

Dr. Joan Giles was a British medical researcher who worked closely with Dr. Saul Krugman on the hepatitis research at Willowbrook State School. While there is less publicly available detailed biographical information about Dr. Giles compared to Dr. Krugman, her contributions to the

---

[13] Maynard, J.E. (1997). The legacy of Saul Krugman. *Hepatology*. 26(3):839–841.

hepatitis studies were significant. Giles, along with Krugman and their team, played a crucial role in conducting the experiments that led to a better understanding of hepatitis transmission and immunity.

Her work at Willowbrook, particularly in the administration and observation of the hepatitis experiments, contributed to the foundational knowledge that paved the way for the development of effective vaccines against hepatitis. Despite the critical role she played in these advancements, Dr. Giles, like Krugman, is also associated with ethical controversies over the use of human subjects in medical research without proper consent.

Despite the many local and national exposés, there is no record of Dr. Saul Krugman or Dr. Joan Giles being formally sanctioned or penalized for their roles in the hepatitis experiments conducted at Willowbrook State School.

The lack of formal sanctions against Dr. Krugman and Dr. Giles highlights the historical context in which these experiments occurred and the evolution of ethical norms and regulations in medical research. The controversy surrounding Willowbrook played a significant role in catalyzing changes in research ethics, including the establishment of Institutional Review Boards (IRBs) and the development of guidelines for informed consent, which are now fundamental components of research involving human subjects.

Drs. Krugman and Giles did not act independently at Willowbrook. Their research received support from several prestigious institutions and entities, including the U.S. Army and the (NIH).[14] These organizations provided funding and resources, facilitating the continuation of the experiments despite ethical concerns. The involvement of such respected bodies lent an air of legitimacy to the research, overshadowing the ethical implications of experimenting on children without their consent.

---

[14] Rothman, D. The Government's Guinea Pigs. https://www.baltimoresun.com/1994/01/11/the-governments-guinea-pigs/ (Accessed 2/2/24).

Ethical Analysis of Experimenting on Mentally Disabled Children

The ethical analysis of the Willowbrook experiments focuses on the violation of consent principles, the exploitation of a vulnerable population, and the conflict of interest inherent in conducting experiments where the well-being of the subjects is secondary to research objectives. The children at Willowbrook, due to their mental disabilities, were unable to consent to participation in the experiments. Consent was often obtained from parents or guardians under the guise of offering admission to Willowbrook — a place where they believed their children would receive care — was contingent upon their child's participation in the experiments, a practice that has been condemned for exploiting the vulnerable population and their families' desperate circumstances. Additionally, the consent signed by parents was worded deceptively. It suggested that the children were receiving a vaccine against the virus rather than being infected with the virus (see footnote 5).

The context in which these decisions were made raises significant ethical questions. Parents were often placed in a difficult position, being told that admission to. This situation blurred the lines between voluntary consent and coercion, compromising the ethical standards of informed consent.

The responsibilities of those making healthcare decisions for the Willowbrook children included ensuring the children's well-being and protecting them from harm. However, the pressure exerted by the research team and the institution itself, coupled with the desperate need for care and support for their children, led many parents to agree to the experiments under duress. This dynamic highlights the ethical responsibility of researchers and institutions to protect vulnerable populations from exploitation, especially in contexts where the ability to give informed consent is compromised.

When questioned about the ethics of these experiments, Krugman and his colleagues argued that the studies were justifiable because they provided valuable insights into the prevention and treatment of hepatitis, and they believed that the children at Willowbrook would have become infected eventually, given the rampant infections that were already present

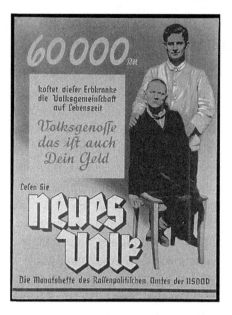

Figure 4.   This poster urges support for Nazi eugenics to control the public expense of sustaining people with genetic disorders. The poster says, "This person who suffers a hereditary disease has a lifelong cost of 60,000 Reichsmarks to the National Community. Fellow German, that is your money as well."

Source: Wiki Commons — Public Domain.

in the institution, suggesting that the life and health of the children at Willowbrook were less important than the goals of his experiments. This is a succinct evocation of the Nazi principle of *Lebensunwertes Leben* or life unworthy of life (Figure 4). A principle that implied that "some people were simply considered disposable."[15]

These experiments have since become a case study in the ethics of medical research, highlighting the importance of informed consent, the protection of vulnerable populations in research, and the necessity of ethical oversight in the conduct of medical experiments.

---

[15] Dr. Stein, S.D. "Life unworthy of life" and other Medical Killing Programes. http://www.ess.uwe.ac.uk/genocide/mord.htm (Accessed 2/21/24).

Long-term Effects and Changes in Research with Vulnerable Populations

The public outcry following the revelation of the Willowbrook experiments led to significant changes in research ethics, particularly concerning vulnerable populations. It catalyzed the development of stricter regulations and oversight mechanisms, including the requirement for informed consent, the establishment of IRBs to review research proposals, and the implementation of ethical guidelines that prioritize the welfare of research subjects over the interests of science or society.

In response to the public outcry, there were significant legal and regulatory responses, primarily focusing on the protection of human subjects in research. These responses helped shape the modern framework of ethical guidelines and regulations governing human subjects research in the United States. The responses included the National Research Act, the Belmont Report, and changes to Federal Regulations for Human Subjects Research (45 CRF 46):

- **National Research Act of 1974**: In response to public outcry over research abuses, including those at Willowbrook, the U.S. Congress passed the National Research Act (Pub. L. No. 93–348) in 1974. This act created the National Commission for the Protection of Human Subjects of Biomedical and Behavioral Research, which was charged with identifying the basic ethical principles that should underlie the conduct of biomedical and behavioral research involving human subjects.[16]

- **The Belmont Report**: Published in 1979 by the National Commission for the Protection of Human Subjects of Biomedical and Behavioral Research, the Belmont Report outlined three fundamental ethical

---

[16]National Commission for the Protection of Human Subjects of Biomedical and Behavioral Research. (1978). *The Belmont Report: Ethical Principles and Guidelines for the Protection of Human Subjects of Research.* Department of Health, Education, and Welfare; National Commission for the Protection of Human Subjects of Biomedical and Behavioral Research. The Belmont Report. Ethical principles and guidelines for the protection of human subjects of research. *J Am Coll Dent.* 2014 Summer; 81(3):4–13.

principles: respect for persons, beneficence, and justice. These principles have since guided the ethical conduct of research involving human subjects in the U.S.

- **Revisions to Federal Regulations for Human Subjects Research (45 CFR 46)**: Following the recommendations of the Belmont Report, federal regulations governing research involving human subjects, known as the Common Rule, were revised to include requirements for informed consent, IRBs, and assurances of compliance by research institutions.[17]

These legal and regulatory responses were direct outcomes of the ethical controversies surrounding research practices at institutions like Willowbrook. They have had a lasting impact on the conduct of research involving human subjects, emphasizing the importance of ethical considerations, participant protection, and oversight.

Conclusion

The hepatitis experiments conducted by Saul Krugman at Willowbrook State School stand as a pivotal moment in the annals of medical ethics. These studies, while contributing significantly to the understanding and management of hepatitis, simultaneously cast a long shadow over the ethical landscape of human research. The controversy that envelops Krugman's work at Willowbrook serves as a stark reminder of the paramount importance of informed consent, the protection of vulnerable populations, and the ethical obligations of researchers. As this chapter closes, it leaves us with an important lesson: the pursuit of scientific knowledge, no matter how noble its intent, must never eclipse the fundamental rights and dignity of the individuals who bear the weight of experimentation. The legacy of Willowbrook, thus, is not solely one of medical advancement but a cautionary tale of the ethical imperatives that must guide all future human research endeavors.

---

[17]Office for Human Research Protections (OHRP). (2009). *45 CFR 46*. https://www.hhs.gov/ohrp/regulations-and-policy/regulations/45-cfr-46/index.html (Accessed 2/2/24).

For Further Reading

1. **"The Willowbrook Wars: Bringing the Mentally Disabled into the Community" by David J. Rothman and Sheila M. Rothman (2005)**
   - This book provides an in-depth look at the Willowbrook State School, detailing the conditions, the hepatitis experiments, and the subsequent legal and ethical battles to reform the institution and protect its residents.
2. **"Human Guinea Pigs: Experimentation on Man" by Maurice Pappworth (1967)**
   - While covering a broader range of human experimentation, Pappworth's work includes a critical examination of the ethical implications of research practices at institutions like Willowbrook.
3. **"Medical Ethics and the Law: Implications for Public Policy" by Milbank Memorial Fund (1980)**
   - This collection of essays and reports touches on the legal and ethical frameworks surrounding medical research, with implications for cases like Willowbrook.
4. **"My Brother's Keeper: A History of the American Association on Intellectual and Developmental Disabilities, 1876–2000" by James W. Conroy and Roberta S. Conroy (2012)**
   - This historical account provides context on the treatment of individuals with intellectual and developmental disabilities in the United States, including the era of Willowbrook.
5. **"No Pity: People with Disabilities Forging a New Civil Rights Movement" by Joseph P. Shapiro (1994)**
   - Shapiro's book discusses the broader civil rights movement for people with disabilities, offering insights into the societal attitudes and policies that impacted institutions like Willowbrook.
6. **"Willowbrook: A Report on How It Is and Why It Doesn't Have to Be That Way" by Geraldo Rivera (1972)**
   - Rivera's investigative report brought national attention to the conditions at Willowbrook, sparking public outrage and calls for reform. This book expands on his findings and the aftermath of the exposé.

7. **"Caring for the Retarded in America: A History" by James W. Trent (1994)**
   - Trent's historical analysis includes discussion of Willowbrook as part of the broader narrative of care for individuals with intellectual disabilities in the United States.
8. **"Mad in America: Bad Science, Bad Medicine, and the Enduring Mistreatment of the Mentally Ill" by Robert Whitaker (2010)**
   - Although focusing on the treatment of mental illness more broadly, Whitaker's book provides context for understanding the systemic issues that allowed places like Willowbrook to exist.
9. **"The State Boys Rebellion" by Michael D'Antonio (2004)**
   - This book tells the story of a group of boys institutionalized in a similar facility to Willowbrook, exploring themes of human rights, experimentation, and the fight for dignity.
10. **"Ethical Considerations in Research on Human Subjects: A Time for Change" by the National Commission for the Protection of Human Subjects of Biomedical and Behavioral Research (1978)**
    - While not exclusively about Willowbrook, this report by the National Commission (which also produced the Belmont Report) addresses the ethical considerations in research that were highlighted by the Willowbrook hepatitis experiments.

Chapter 5

An Examination of Radiation Experiments

In the annals of American history, the radiation experiments conducted on disabled people in the mid-20th century stand as glaring reminders of a period marked by egregious ethical lapses in scientific research. These experiments, which involved the deliberate exposure of unsuspecting populations to radioactive substances, epitomize the profound abuse of vulnerable subjects under the guise of national security and scientific advancement.

In Massachusetts, researchers, sponsored by Quaker Oats cereal company, encouraged intellectually disabled children to eat bowls of cereal with radioactive iron and calcium in it, to analyze the distribution of these elements in the human body and ascertain the health benefits of the sponsor's oatmeal.

In Cincinnati, researchers at the University of Cincinnati exposed terminally ill patients, to high doses of radiation to observe its effects on the human body.

In addition to the aforementioned experiments, the Alaskan Iodine-131 experiments represent another significant instance of radiation research involving vulnerable populations. Conducted in remote Alaskan villages, these experiments involved the administration of radioactive Iodine-131 to indigenous populations to study thyroid function and the potential effects of radiation exposure. The selection of these communities and the lack of informed consent or clear communication of the research's nature

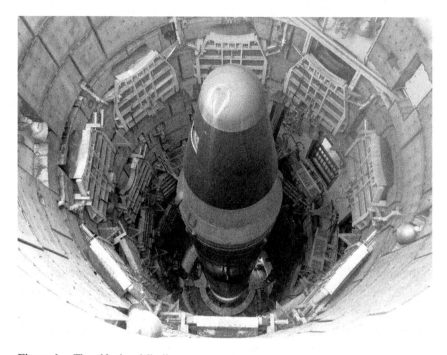

Figure 1.   Titan Nuclear Missile.
Source: Mike McBey Wiki commons CC by 2.0.

and risks highlight the ethical breaches that characterized radiation experiments of the era. These studies aimed to gather data relevant to understanding how radiation exposure could affect thyroid health, particularly in the context of nuclear fallout. However, like other mid-20th-century radiation experiments, they raise profound ethical concerns about the exploitation of marginalized populations for scientific research.

The Cincinnati prisoner experiments, the Fernald State School experiments, and the Alaskan Radioactive iodine experiments were all conducted in a social and political environment shaped by several key factors, including the Cold War, the race for nuclear supremacy, and a less developed framework for research ethics. This context stimulated the perceived need for these studies, reflecting broader societal and governmental priorities of the time (Figure 1).

The Cold War (approximately 1947–1991) between the United States and the Soviet Union was a period of intense ideological conflict and competition, including the nuclear arms race. Both superpowers sought to develop and expand their nuclear arsenals, leading to a heightened focus on understanding the effects of radiation exposure. The fear of nuclear warfare and the potential need to protect or treat the population in the event of a nuclear incident drove much of the interest in radiation research. This urgency justified, in the eyes of some researchers and government officials, the use of vulnerable populations in experiments without adequate informed consent.[1,2]

During the mid-20th century, the ethical standards governing human subjects research were not as developed or universally enforced as they are today. The Nuremberg Code was established in 1947, setting forth principles for ethical medical research, including the necessity of voluntary consent.[3] However, these principles were not fully integrated into U.S. research practices until much later. This gap allowed researchers and government agencies to conduct experiments on human subjects without the stringent ethical oversight that would be required today.

The choice of subjects for these experiments — prisoners, minorities, children with intellectual disabilities, and poor urban populations — reflects societal attitudes of racism and classism that devalued the rights and autonomy of these groups.[4] These populations were seen as convenient subjects for research that would be considered too risky or unethical for more privileged members of society. There was a pervasive belief that the contributions of such experiments to science and national security justified the risks imposed on the subjects.

The social and political environment that stimulated the need for the Cincinnati prisoner experiments and the Fernald State School experiments was characterized by a confluence of Cold War imperatives, nascent research ethics, societal attitudes that marginalized certain populations,

---

[1] Jonathan, D.M. (1999). *Undue Risk: Secret State Experiments on Humans.* W. H. Freeman; 1st edition (September 11, 1999).

[2] Eileen, W. (1999). *The Plutonium Files: America's Secret Medical Experiments in the Cold War.* The Dial Press; 1st edition.

[3] Shuster, E. (1997). Fifty years later: The significance of the Nuremberg code. *New England Journal of Medicine.* 337(20):1436–1440. doi: 10.1056/NEJM199711133372006. PMID 9358142. S2CID 9950045.

[4] Reverby, S.M. (1978). Racism and Research: The Case of the Tuskegee Syphilis Study. *Hastings Center Report.* 8(6):21–29.

and strong governmental and institutional support for scientific and military advancements. This context facilitated the conduct of research that, by today's standards, represents significant ethical violations, highlighting the importance of ethical vigilance and the protection of vulnerable populations in research.

Responsible for these experiments were a coalition of scientists, physicians, and military officials, each bringing their expertise and interests to the table. The experiments were supported by a mix of federal and military funding, with significant contributions from the Atomic Energy Commission (AEC) and the Department of Defense (DoD), reflecting the national security implications of the research. These entities were deeply invested in understanding radiation's biological effects, aiming to develop protective measures for military personnel and assess the feasibility of using radiation in warfare scenarios.

Institutions like universities and state schools played roles in facilitating the research, too. They were encouraged by the promise of scientific advancement, prestige, and government funding.

The choice to conduct these experiments was driven by the urgent need for empirical data on radiation's effects on human health. In the aftermath of World War II and the onset of the Cold War, the potential for nuclear conflict loomed large, making this research seem imperative for national defense.

Following extensive research, the Soviet Union successfully developed its nuclear arsenal in 1949, marking the beginning of a period throughout the Cold War where the specter of nuclear conflict was a constant concern. Particularly in the United States, the apprehension of a nuclear apocalypse was widespread, leading to the construction of bunkers in communities and the institution of "duck and cover" exercises for students across multiple generations in schools.[5]

---

[5]The university of Kansas, Center for Russian, East European and Eurasian Studies. https://coldwarheartland.ku.edu/legacies/united-states#:~:text=After%20years%20of%20 research%2C%20the,and%20cover%E2%80%9D%20drills%20in%20school (Accessed 2/20/24).

Additionally, the medical community's growing interest in radiation as a therapeutic tool necessitated a deeper understanding of its biological impacts to optimize treatment protocols and minimize harm to patients.[6]

One notable example of these experiments involved the exposure of cancer patients to varying levels of radiation to observe its therapeutic effects and document potential side effects.[7] While these studies contributed valuable data to the field of oncology, they also raised ethical concerns, particularly regarding the adequacy of informed consent and the selection of subjects. Many of the patients involved were from vulnerable populations, including those with limited access to healthcare or understanding of the risks involved, highlighting significant ethical lapses in the conduct of the research.

Within the broader scope of radiation experiments conducted in the mid-20th century, a notable series focused on the use of radioactive iodine, particularly Iodine-131. This isotope was selected for its medical applications in diagnosing and treating thyroid conditions, leveraging its ability to concentrate in the thyroid gland, thereby providing valuable diagnostic information and therapeutic benefits. However, the ethical boundaries of medical research were significantly breached when Iodine-131 was administered to individuals without a clear therapeutic rationale or without proper disclosure that it was part of a research study.

These experiments, therefore, represent a complex interplay of scientific ambition, medical advancement, and military preparedness, underscored by troubling ethical oversights. The legacy of these experiments continues to inform contemporary debates on the ethics of human subject research, emphasizing the need for rigorous informed consent processes and the protection of participants from harm.

---

[6] Gianfaldoni, S., Gianfaldoni, R., Wollina, U., Lotti, J., Tchernev, G. and Lotti, T. (2017). An overview on radiotherapy: From Its history to its current applications in dermatology. *Open Access Maced J Med Sci.* 5(4):521–525. doi: 10.3889/oamjms.2017.122.

[7] Eileen, W. (1999). *The Plutonium Files: America's Secret Medical Experiments in the Cold War.* The Dial Press; 1st edition.

The Experiments at Fernald State School

The Walter E. Fernald Developmental Center, originally named the Massachusetts School for the Feeble-Minded, was the Western Hemisphere's oldest publicly funded institution serving people with developmental disabilities. Located in Waltham, Massachusetts, it was founded in the mid-19th century and named after Walter E. Fernald, a prominent advocate of eugenics and the institution's first resident superintendent who served from 1887. This center was involved in several experiments that used residents as test subjects. These experiments were part of a broader series of studies aimed at understanding the nutritional and metabolic effects of radioactive substances in the human body. These studies were spearheaded by researchers from the Massachusetts Institute of Technology (MIT) and sponsored by Quaker Oats, in collaboration with the Atomic Energy Commission (AEC).

In 1956, MIT Professor of Nutrition Robert S. Harris led the experiment, which studied the absorption of calcium and iron. He and fellow researchers at the Fernald School gave mentally disabled children radioactive calcium orally. In the 1940s and 1950s, more than 100 boys were fed oatmeal laced with radioactive iron and calcium in an experiment to show the nutritional value of Quaker Oats cereals. The primary objective was to investigate how the body absorbs nutrients from food and to compare the nutritional value of different cereals, specifically Quaker oatmeal versus Cream of Wheat.

The most controversial aspect of these experiments involved feeding the boys oatmeal mixed with radioactive iron (Fe-59) and calcium (Ca-45) tracers. These isotopes were chosen because they could be easily detected in the body, allowing researchers to track the absorption and metabolism of iron and calcium from the oatmeal.

In addition to the contaminated food, some experiments involved directly injecting subjects with radioactive calcium. This method was intended to provide a clearer understanding of calcium metabolism, bypassing the digestive process to see how the body handles calcium directly introduced into the bloodstream.

The boys at Fernald who participated in these studies were not informed of the radioactive nature of the oatmeal or injections. They were chosen because they were considered a convenient sample group, living in a controlled environment where their diet and health could be monitored closely. The lack of informed consent and the selection of a vulnerable population for these experiments are among the most significant ethical concerns raised by these studies.

The administration of radioactive substances without informed consent led to potential health risks for the subjects, including increased risk of cancer and other radiation-induced diseases. The long-term health effects of these exposures were often not tracked, leaving unanswered questions about the full impact on the participants' health.

The revelation of these experiments in the 1990s led to public outcry and a reevaluation of ethical standards in scientific research. A 1995 class-action lawsuit filed by former Fernald students against MIT and Quaker Oats resulted in a 1998 District court decision awarding the victims a $1.85 million settlement from MIT and Quaker.[8] This settlement highlighted the need for greater protection for research subjects, especially those who are vulnerable or incapable of giving informed consent. Indeed, the Fernald experiments contributed to the tightening of regulations governing human subjects research in the United States. The National Research Act of 1974, which established the National Commission for the Protection of Human Subjects of Biomedical and Behavioral Research, and the development of Institutional Review Boards (IRBs) were part of the response to such ethical violations. These bodies are tasked with reviewing and approving research involving human subjects to ensure that studies are ethical and that participants are fully informed and consent to the research.

In 1994, the MIT task force found that "although the research was conducted in violation of the fundamental human rights of the subjects involved" the exposure to these radioactive tracers caused "no significant health effects."[9,10]

---

[8] Hussain, Zareena (January 7, 1998). MIT to pay $1.85 million in Fernald radiation settlement. *The Tech*. Vol. 11, no. 65. Archived from the original on June 21, 2009 (Accessed 2/23/24).

[9] MIT News. Task force finds Fernald research had no significant health effects https://news.mit.edu/1994/fernald-0511 (Accessed 2/3/24).

[10] "Chapter 7: The Studies at Fernald School". *ACHRE Report. It is clear that the doses involved were low and that it is extremely unlikely that any of the children who were used as subjects were harmed as a consequence.*

The experiments conducted at the Fernald State School serve as a reminder about the ethical considerations necessary in scientific research. They underscore the importance of informed consent, the protection of vulnerable populations, and the need for oversight to prevent the exploitation of research subjects. The legacy of these experiments has shaped the ethical frameworks that govern human subjects research today, ensuring that the rights and welfare of participants are a paramount concern.

The institutions involved in these experiments, including MIT and the AEC, bear a significant portion of the responsibility for the ethical violations that occurred. Researchers and administrators at these institutions either overlooked or dismissed the ethical implications of conducting experiments on vulnerable populations without proper consent. The lack of transparency and the guise of medical treatment under which these studies were conducted represent a profound ethical failure.

Cincinnati Radiation Experiments

The Cincinnati Radiation Experiments, conducted from 1960 to 1971 at the Cincinnati General Hospital (now the University of Cincinnati Hospital), represent a dark and controversial chapter in the history of medical research in the United States. Under the leadership of radiologist Eugene L. Saenger (Figure 2) and funded in part by the Defense Atomic Support Agency of the DoD, these experiments aimed to uncover the effects of significant radiation exposure on soldiers during nuclear conflict.[11,12] They subjected at least 90 patients with advanced cancer to total and partial body irradiation. The experiments were marked by ethical breaches, including the lack of informed consent and the severe adverse effects experienced by participants. The experiments ended in 1972 amidst growing scrutiny and were later thrust back into the public eye,

---

[11] United States. Advisory Committee on Human Radiation Experiments (1996). *The Human Radiation Experiments*. USA: Oxford University Press. pp. 239–240.

[12] Stephens, M. (2002). *The Treatment: The Story of Those Who Died in the Cincinnati Radiation Tests*. Durham and London: Duke University Press. pp. 3–14.

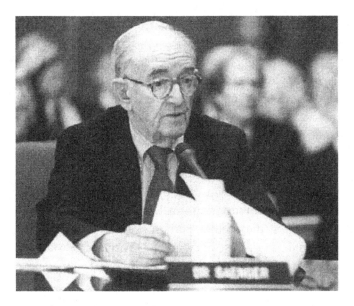

Figure 2. Eugene L. Saenger, MD.
Source: Marshall Thomas photographer.

leading to significant legal and ethical repercussions. This chapter delves into the complex narrative of the Cincinnati Radiation Experiments, exploring the motivations behind them, the experiences of the patients involved, and the lasting impact on ethical standards in human research.

Dr. Saenger, like many other researchers mentioned in this book, was an ambitious and hardworking scientist who came from a privileged background. He graduated from Harvard University and the Cincinnati College of Medicine. He was an eminent figure in the field of radiology and director of the university's radioisotope laboratory when he began these experiments.[13]

Dr. Saenger aimed to explore a critical question for the Pentagon during the Cold War: how much radiation could a soldier endure without suffering disorientation or incapacitation?[14] His experiments, conducted under a

---

[13] Thomas H.M. (October 6, 2007). Eugene Saenger, 90; pioneer in radiation research, *Los Angeles Times*.

[14] United States. Advisory Committee on Human Radiation Experiments (1996). *The Human Radiation Experiments*. USA: Oxford University Press. pp. 239–240.

contract with the Department of Defense (DoD), were specifically designed to assess the cognitive and physiological impacts of radiation on soldiers.[15] These tests were supported by the Cincinnati General Hospital, the University of Cincinnati, and the US Defense Department. The Defense Department alone spent $651,000 to support the Cincinnati experiments (see footnote 9).

To mimic the conditions a soldier might face, patients were positioned in defensive postures before being subjected to high doses of whole-body radiation. This approach allowed for the observation of their physical and mental reactions in real time.[16] Unlike the standard medical practice of the era, which involved administering small, cumulative doses of radiation to cancer patients for therapeutic purposes, these experiments exposed patients to a single, large dose of radiation.[17] This method starkly contrasts with Dr. Saenger's later claims that the experiments had therapeutic intentions for the patients.[18]

The process entailed a single administration of 25–300 rads of Cobalt-60 radiation to patients,[19] equivalent to the radiation from 20,000 chest X-rays.[20] This intense dosage resulted in severe side effects for 48 out of 88 patients, including nausea, vomiting, diarrhea, loss of appetite, abdominal pain, severe weight loss, bleeding, hallucinations, and confusion.[21] A 1972 study by three junior faculty members at the University of

---

[15] Egilman, D. (1998). *A Little Too Much of the Buchenwald Touch? Military Radiation Research at the University of Cincinnati, 1960–1972.* India: Overseas Publishers Association. p. 69.

[16] Stephens, M. (2002). *The Treatment: The Story of Those Who Died in the Cincinnati Radiation Tests.* Durham and London: Duke University Press. pp. 3–14.

[17] Egilman, D. (1998). *A Little Too Much of the Buchenwald Touch? Military Radiation Research at the University of Cincinnati, 1960–1972.* India: Overseas Publishers Association. p. 70.

[18] Saenger, E. (2002). *Hearing Testimony of Eugene Saenger.* Durham and London: Duke University Press. pp. 296–305.

[19] Stephens, M. (2002). *The Treatment: The Story of Those Who Died in the Cincinnati Radiation Tests.* Durham and London: Duke University Press. p. 180.

[20] Stephens, M. (2002). *The Treatment: The Story of Those Who Died in the Cincinnati Radiation Tests.* Durham and London. Duke University Press. p. 180.

[21] Schneider, K. (1994-04-11). Cold war radiation test on humans to undergo a congressional review. *The New York Times.* Retrieved 2017-04-30.

Cincinnati suggested that up to a quarter of these patients might have died from the radiation exposure itself rather than their underlying cancer.[22] Within two months of receiving the radiation, about 25% of the patients passed away, and the first year saw the death of more than 75% of them.[23]

The subjects of the experiment were at least 89 cancer patients, ranging in age from 9 to 84, most of whom were terminally ill and poor, and 60% of whom were black.[24] All the patients had advanced-stage disease[25] but were otherwise in good nutritional health.[26] The Cincinnati General Hospital's Tumor Clinic referred the patients to Dr. Saenger's care.[27] While the average age of the patients was 59 years, this group also included three children who were 9, 10, and 13 years old.[28]

Despite the suffering and potential harm, most patients did not start signing consent forms until 1965,[29] and even then, they were not informed of the Pentagon's involvement or the experiment's full risks.[30] This was despite the requirements of informed consent demanded by the Cincinnati General Hospital; the Department of Health, Education, and Welfare; and

---

[22] https://www.nytimes.com/1994/04/11/us/cold-war-radiation-test-on-humans-to-undergo-a-congressional-review.html (Accessed 2/21/24).

[23] Saenger, E. (2002). *Hearing Testimony of Eugene Saenger.* Durham and London. Duke University Press. pp. 296–305.

[24] Stephens, M. (2002). *The Treatment: The Story of Those Who Died in the Cincinnati Radiation Tests.* Durham and London: Duke University Press. pp. 293–295.

[25] *Ibid.*

[26] Egilman, D. (1998). *A Little Too Much of the Buchenwald Touch? Military Radiation Research at the University of Cincinnati, 1960–1972.* India: Overseas Publishers Association. p. 72.

[27] Saenger, E. (2002). *Hearing Testimony of Eugene Saenger.* Durham and London: Duke University Press. pp. 296–305.

[28] Egilman, D. (1998). *A Little Too Much of the Buchenwald Touch? Military Radiation Research at the University of Cincinnati, 1960–1972.* India: Overseas Publishers Association. p. 73.

[29] Egilman, D. (1998). *A Little Too Much of the Buchenwald Touch? Military Radiation Research at the University of Cincinnati, 1960–1972.* India: Overseas Publishers Association. p. 77.

[30] Stephens, M. (2002). *The Treatment: The Story of Those Who Died in the Cincinnati Radiation Tests.* Durham and London: Duke University Press. p. 10.

the DoD.[31] This lack of informed consent and the concealment of the experiment's true nature and risks highlight significant ethical lapses by the researchers.

In 1969, after the National Institutes of Health reviewed the ethical practices at Cincinnati General Hospital, Dr. Saenger introduced a revised consent form (see footnote 9). This new form provided patients with details about the purpose, procedures, and risks associated with the irradiation tests. However, it notably did not mention the possibility of death as a risk.[32]

The revelations of these experiments have led to legal and regulatory scrutiny, including lawsuits against Dr. Saenger, his colleagues, and the university by the families of some patients. Congressional hearings were called to investigate the matter further, revealing internal disagreements and criticisms within the University of Cincinnati about the experiment's safety and morality. Senator Ted Kennedy began an inquiry and wanted to interview the surviving patients exposed to radiation in this experiment, which Dr. Saenger resisted.[33] In April 1972, Senator Kennedy, Ohio Governor John Gilligan, and Warren Bennis, who was the president of the University of Cincinnati at the time, came to an agreement. Rather than imposing fines and imprisoning the researchers, they decided to stop the political investigations into the Cincinnati Radiation Experiments on the condition that the contract linking UC researchers with the DoD was ended.[34] As a result of this agreement, a full inquiry into the experiments was never completed, and Dr. Saenger's reputation remained largely intact, later, he even received a gold medal for "career achievements" from the Radiological Society of North America.[35]

---

[31] Saenger, E. (2002). Op cit.

[32] Stephens, M. (2002). *The Treatment: The Story of Those Who Died in the Cincinnati Radiation Tests.* Durham and London: Duke University Press. p. 17.

[33] Stephens, M. (2002). *The Treatment: The Story of Those Who Died in the Cincinnati Radiation Tests.* Durham and London: Duke University Press. p. 12.

[34] United States. Advisory Committee on Human Radiation Experiments (1996). *The Human Radiation Experiments.* USA: Oxford University Press. pp. 240.

[35] Dicke, W. Eugene Saenger, Controversial Doctor, Dies at 90. *The New York Times.* Retrieved 29 April 2016.

The families of the patients in these experiments filed a lawsuit alleging that the patient's rights had been violated by concealing the true nature of the experiments and the risks involved.[36] Eventually, the case was settled for over $4 million, which was paid for by the University of Cincinnati, the City of Cincinnati, and the individual researchers.[37,38]

The ethical lapses in this case include the failure to obtain informed consent, the exposure of patients to harmful procedures without clear therapeutic benefits, and the concealment of the experiment's military purposes from the subjects. These lapses have contributed to an ongoing debate about the ethics of human experimentation and the need for greater transparency and protection for research subjects.

The Holmesburg Prison Experiments: A Dark Chapter in Medical Research

The Holmesburg Prison experiments, a series of medical tests conducted on inmates, represent one of the most controversial episodes in the history of American medical research.[39] These experiments took place primarily during the 1950s through the 1970s at Holmesburg Prison in Philadelphia, Pennsylvania. This period was marked by a burgeoning interest in advancing medical and dermatological knowledge, often at the expense of ethical considerations. The Cold War era, with its emphasis on scientific progress and national security, created a backdrop that encouraged risky medical experiments, including those involving radioactive substances.

Several social forces encouraged these experiments. The era's scientific optimism, combined with a lack of stringent ethical oversight, created an environment where the ends of medical advancement seemingly justified the means. Additionally, the prison population was viewed as a

---

[36] Hawk, M.L. (1995). *The "Kingdom of Ends": In Re Cincinnati Radiation Litigation and the Right to Bodily Integrity.* Cas. W. Res. L. Rev. 977.

[37] Stephens, M. (2002). *The Treatment: The Story of Those Who Died in the Cincinnati Radiation Tests.* Durham and London: Duke University Press. pp. xxi.

[38] Peggy O'Farrell. Radiology guru Saenger dies. *The Cincinnati Enquirer.*

[39] Ex-Holmesburg Inmates File Suit Over Experiments, *The Philadelphia Inquirer.* Philadelphia, Pennsylvania. October 18, 2000. Retrieved November 9, 2009.

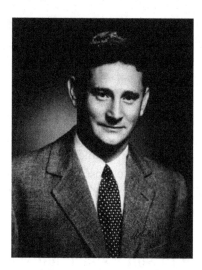

Figure 3.   Albert Kligman, MD.
Source: Image from the National Library of Medicine.

convenient and cost-effective resource for medical research, reflecting societal attitudes that devalued the rights and dignity of incarcerated individuals.

The most prominent researcher associated with the Holmesburg experiments was Dr. Albert M. Kligman (Figure 3).[40] Kligman was born to Jewish immigrant parents in Philadelphia on March 17, 1916.[41] He pursued his education at the University of Pennsylvania, earning a bachelor's degree in 1939 and a Doctorate in botany three years later. In 1947, Kligman completed his Medical Degree at the same university and chose dermatology as his specialty, applying his expertise in fungal studies.

Kligman's motivation stemmed from a desire to advance dermatological science and, arguably, personal ambition. At the time, Kligman's attitude toward the subjects of his experiments could be summed up in his remarks about the prisoners in Holmesburg, an "idle collection of

---

[40] Gellene, D. (2010). Dr. Albert M. Kligman, Dermatologist, Dies at 93. *The New York Times*. Retrieved 2/4/24.

[41] Gellene, D (2010). *Op cit.*

humanity that seemed ideal for dermatologic study."[42] When recounting his first visit to Holmesburg Prison, he stated, "All I saw before me were acres of skin. It was like a farmer seeing a fertile field for the first time."[43]

His work at Holmesburg led to significant developments, including the discovery of Retin-A, a widely used acne treatment. However, the means by which these discoveries were made have overshadowed his scientific contributions.

These experiments were sponsored and supported by a range of entities, including the U.S. military, pharmaceutical companies, chemical companies, and the University of Pennsylvania. The military's interest lay in understanding the effects of radiation and chemical warfare agents on human health, while pharmaceutical companies sought to test the efficacy and safety of various products. The University of Pennsylvania, through its association with Kligman, provided the institutional backing necessary to conduct these experiments.

Dr. Albert Kligman's research on inmates was notably extensive and controversial, involving exposure to a wide array of harmful substances including herpes virus, staphylococcus, cosmetics, skin-blistering chemicals, radioactive isotopes, psychoactive drugs, and carcinogens like dioxins. His work was supported financially by 33 different entities, among them Johnson & Johnson, Dow Chemicals, and the U.S. Army.

The specifics of these experiments, including the outcomes and long-term health impacts on the participants, have been difficult to fully ascertain due to the secretive nature of the research and the lack of comprehensive follow-up with the subjects. However, patient reports allow inmates subjected to these experiments to face severe treatments. One reported exposure to microwave radiation and corrosive acids that transformed forearm skin to a leather-like texture and caused blistering in sensitive areas.[44] Beyond chemical exposure, inmates underwent physical

---

[42] Hornblum, A. (2000). Subjected to medical experimentation: Pennsylvania's contribution to 'science' in prisons. *Pennsylvania History*, 67(3): 415–426.

[43] Meyer, C.R. (1999). Unwitting consent: 'Acres of Skin: Human Experiments at Holmesburg Prison' tells the story of medical researchers who sacrificed the rights of their subjects for personal profit. *Minnesota Medicine*, 82(7): 53–54.

[44] Hornblum, A.M. (1998). *Acres of Skin: Human Experiments at Holmesburg Prison: A True Story of Abuse and Exploitation in the Name of Medical Science*. Routledge.

exertion followed by surgical removal of sweat glands for analysis. In more harrowing instances, cadaver fragments were implanted into inmates to test for organ regeneration. A former inmate expressed the dehumanizing nature of these experiments, stating, "They used my body; they did things to me that were inhuman... . I feel less than a woman because of the things they did to me. This brought me pain. A lot of pain."[45] The experiments extended beyond individual harm, affecting the health of entire cell blocks with the spread of biological agents like the Hong Kong flu, poison ivy, and poison oak.[46] It was estimated that 80–90% of the inmates in a 1,200-person prison facility were subjected to experimentation.[47]

The motivation for the prisoners to participate in these experiments was two-fold. They could earn money and shorten their sentences. The Holmesburg Prison experiments offered compensation ranging from $30 to $50, and in some cases, up to $800, which was significantly higher than what other prison jobs paid. At that time in Philadelphia's prisons, inmates had the option to shorten their sentences by paying 10% of their bail amount.[46] This made participating in experiments a viable way for inmates to quickly earn the necessary funds for their release.

The radiation experiments at Holmesburg Prison are believed to have involved exposing inmates to ionizing radiation to study its effects on human skin and the body's overall response. These studies were likely motivated by the military's interest in understanding how to treat or prevent radiation sickness in the event of nuclear warfare. The specifics of the dosage, duration, and exact nature of the radioactive materials used are not widely detailed in public records. However, the overarching concern was the potential for these exposures to increase the risk of cancer and other serious health conditions in the subjects.

Similarly, chemical warfare experiments conducted on Holmesburg inmates involved the application or exposure to chemical agents that could

---

[45] Holmesburg Experiments. *Exploiting Humans for Medical Research.* https:// humanmedicalresearch.weebly.com/holmesburg-experiments.html Retrieved 2/21/24.
[46] Hornblum, A.M. (1998). *Acres of Skin: Human Experiments at Holmesburg Prison: A True Story of Abuse and Exploitation in the Name of Medical Science.* Routledge.
[47] Hornblum, A. (2007). *Sentenced to Science: One black man's story of imprisonment in America.* University Park: Pennsylvania State UP.

be used in military contexts. One of the most notorious of these involved the use of dioxin, a highly toxic compound known to be a contaminant in the herbicide Agent Orange, used by the U.S. military during the Vietnam War.[48] Inmates were exposed to dioxin and other chemicals to observe the skin's reaction and the potential systemic effects, without proper informed consent or adequate safety measures in place. Inmates were subjected to injections of pesticides to determine safe dosage levels. Unfortunately, these experiments often involved administering doses that led to severe side effects, including chloracne, inflammatory pustules, and papules, with symptoms persisting for 4–7 months. The usual caution and conservatism that surround medical research were abandoned. Remarkably, more than 10 participants received over 7,500 micrograms of dioxin pesticide, a quantity that astonished even the scientists at Dow Chemical (see footnote 46). As the experiments progressed, the dosages escalated to 468 times higher than the initially suggested safe amounts.

Both sets of experiments raised significant ethical and health concerns. Participants often experienced immediate adverse effects, such as skin irritation, burns, and rashes. The long-term implications, including the potential for developing cancers or other serious health conditions, have been a source of ongoing concern and debate. The lack of transparency and the failure to fully inform participants of the risks represent grave ethical violations, contributing to the legacy of Holmesburg as a symbol of the darkest aspects of medical research ethics.

The subjects in these experiments were inmates at Holmesburg Prison, many of whom were African Americans.[49] These men were induced to participate through financial incentives, offering a way to earn money in an environment where opportunities to do so were scarce. The promise of minor compensation appealed to many inmates, especially those with few external support systems.

Participants were often inadequately informed about the experiments' risks and benefits. In many cases, the true nature of the substances applied or administered, including radioactive materials, was not disclosed. The

---

[48] Epstein, A (1981). Human Guinea Pigs: Dioxin Tested at Holmesburg, Philadelphia Inquirer.
[49] Hornblum, A.M. (1998). *Acres of Skin: Human Experiments at Holmesburg Prison.*

consent obtained from these inmates was questionable at best, given the power dynamics and the lack of comprehensive information provided about the potential dangers involved.

Many of the subjects experienced adverse reactions ranging from skin rashes and burns to more severe health issues. The use of radioactive substances and other hazardous materials raised significant concerns about the long-term health effects on participants, including the potential for increased cancer risk, though direct links to deaths are less clearly documented in public sources.

Ethical lapses

The ethical lapses in the Holmesburg experiments were profound, including the following.

The ethical analysis of Dr. Albert Kligman's experiments at Holmesburg Prison reveals significant breaches of ethical principles that guide human research. These experiments, which involved exposing inmates to a variety of harmful substances, including dioxins and other toxic chemicals, raise profound ethical concerns:

1. **Informed Consent**: A cornerstone of ethical research, informed consent, was notably absent or inadequately obtained in Kligman's experiments. The inmates were often not fully informed about the risks and nature of the experiments, undermining their autonomy and ability to make an informed decision about participation.

2. **Exploitation of Vulnerable Populations**: The selection of prison inmates as subjects exploited a vulnerable population. Inmates, due to their incarceration, have limited freedom and may feel coerced into participating in research, especially when financial compensation is involved.[50] This dynamic creates an inherently coercive environment, compromising the voluntariness of their consent.

3. **Risk vs. Benefit**: Ethical research mandates that the risks to subjects must be minimized and balanced against the potential benefits.

---

[50] Philadelphia's Abandoned Holmesburg Prison: A Dream of Release. *www.abandone damerica.us*. Retrieved 2/2/2024.

Kligman's experiments subjected inmates to significant health risks, including the development of chloracne and other severe conditions, without clear benefits to the participants. The primary beneficiaries of the research were the sponsoring entities, including pharmaceutical and chemical companies, and not the subjects themselves.

4. **Justice**: The principle of justice requires the equitable selection of research subjects. Kligman's focus on inmates concentrated the research risks on a socially and economically disadvantaged group, while the benefits of the research extended to broader society, violating this principle.

5. **Respect for Persons**: This principle encompasses treating individuals as autonomous agents and protecting those with diminished autonomy. Kligman's experiments failed to respect the personhood of the inmates by using them as means to an end rather than respecting their inherent dignity and rights.

Kligman's Holmesburg Prison experiments represent a stark violation of ethical standards in research. The lack of informed consent, exploitation of a vulnerable population, disproportionate risk without benefit to the subjects, injustice in subject selection, and failure to respect the autonomy and dignity of the inmates highlight the ethical lapses of these experiments. These violations underscore the importance of ethical oversight in research to protect the rights and well-being of participants.

The ethical lapses and the physical harm inflicted upon the inmates have been well documented and criticized, leading to significant changes in regulations governing human subject research.[51] However, the full extent of the harm, including mortality, remains a subject of investigation and debate. The lack of transparency and accountability at the time of the experiments has made it difficult to fully assess the impact on the health and mortality of the participants.

---

[51] Hornblum, A.M. (1999) Ethical Lapses in Dermatologic "Research". *Arch Dermatol.* 135(4):383–385. doi: 10.1001/archderm.135.4.383.

Revelations

The revelation of the ethical lapses in the Holmesburg experiments and others like them led to significant public outcry and a reevaluation of ethical standards in medical research.[52]

The Kligman experiments at Holmesburg Prison became widely known to the public in the early 1970s through investigative journalism and public scrutiny. The ethical issues surrounding these experiments were exposed in detail when Allen M. Hornblum published his book *Acres of Skin* in 1998. Hornblum's work brought significant attention to the experiments, highlighting the exploitation and ethical violations involved in Kligman's research on incarcerated men. This publication played a crucial role in raising awareness about the experiments and their impact on the inmates involved.

Regulatory changes, including the establishment of IRBs and the implementation of federal regulations governing human subjects research, were instituted to prevent such abuses in the future. The National Research Act of 1974 and the Belmont Report of 1979 laid the groundwork for these reforms, emphasizing the importance of informed consent, the assessment of risks and benefits, and the selection of subjects. In 1976, the National Commission for the Protection of Human Subjects of Biomedical and Behavioral Research passed a regulation protecting prisoners from unethical research practices.[53] This was largely due to Klignman's prison research.[54] Human experimentation in prisons effectively came to an end in the US a few years after the commission made these recommendations.

The Holmesburg Prison experiments serve as a cautionary tale about the dangers of prioritizing scientific advancement over ethical considerations. While the regulatory landscape has since evolved to protect research subjects better, the legacy of Holmesburg remains a vivid reminder of the need for vigilance and ethical integrity in medical research.

---

[52] Wolfgang, W. Medical experiments on humans and the development of guidelines governing them: the central role of dermatology. *Clinics in Dermatology*, 27(4), 384–394.

[53] The Advisory Committee on Human Radiation Experiments Final Report, U.S. Government Printing Office, Pg 422.

[54] Human Subjects Timeline – Office of NIH History and Stetten Museum. https://history.nih.gov/display/history/Human+Subjects+Timeline (Accessed 2/21/24).

Albert Kligman and others involved in these experiments were never formally sanctioned. One of his experiments in Holmesburg Prison led to the identification of the use of tretinoin as a treatment for acne and wrinkles. Sold as Retin-A, this innovation earned Kligman significant royalties. Although several former prisoners attempted to sue Dr. Kligman and the University of Pennsylvania for intent to harm.[55] The lawsuit was dismissed because it was filed after the statute of limitations had expired. He died of coronary artery disease in February 2010, at age 93.[56]

The Iodine-131 Experiments in Alaska

The Alaskan Iodine-131 (I-131) study, conducted by the Arctic Aeromedical Laboratory (AAL) in the 1950s, was part of a broader effort to understand human acclimatization to cold environments. The study involved administering I131, a radioactive tracer, to measure thyroid function in both Alaska Natives and white military personnel. The research aimed to explore the role of the thyroid in adapting to cold temperatures, with the hypothesis that the thyroid might play a significant role in this process. The study was conducted under the guidelines provided by the U.S. AEC, with Dr. Kaare Rodahl (Figure 4) leading the project after completing the required training in radioisotope usage and methods.

The AAL study included Alaska Natives from various villages (such as Wainwright, Point Lay, Anaktuvuk Pass, Fort Yukon, Arctic Village, and Point Hope) and white military personnel. Subjects were chosen based on their availability and willingness to participate. In the case of Alaska Natives, village elders were approached, and the purpose of the study was explained to them. The elders then communicated with their community members and helped in recruiting volunteers. For military personnel, volunteers were sought through announcements made by commanding officers.

---

[55]Ly Bck, Eb D, Jl F *et al.* (2021) Reconsidering Named Honorifics in Medicine—the Troubling Legacy of Dermatologist Albert Kligman. *JAMA Dermatology.* 157(2):153–155.
[56]Albert M. Kligman, dermatologist who patented Retin-A, dies at 93. https://www.washingtonpost.com/wp-dyn/content/article/2010/02/21/AR2010022104116.htmls (Accessed 2/21/24).

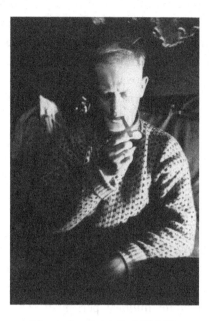

Figure 4.   Kaare Rodahl, MD.

The study population included Alaskan natives and white military personnel. The Alaska Native participants included 102 individuals from various villages across northern and central Alaska. The study involved both men and women, including individuals of childbearing age and some who were lactating. The ages of the Alaska Native participants ranged from 16 to 90 years old. The villages visited for the study included Wainwright, Point Lay, Anaktuvuk Pass, Fort Yukon, Arctic Village, and Point Hope. The selection of these villages was based on their geographical location and the living conditions that exposed residents to extreme cold, making them ideal subjects for studying acclimatization to the Arctic environment.

The study also included 19 white servicemen from the U.S. Air Force and Army stationed in Fairbanks, Alaska. These participants were all male, with ages ranging from 19 to 37 years. The inclusion of military personnel was aimed at comparing the thyroid activity and acclimatization processes between individuals accustomed to the Arctic environment (Alaska Natives) and those who were not (military personnel).

The AAL Technical Report[57] identified two subjects from Wainwright and one subject from Arctic Village who were nursing children at the time of their participation in the study. Since radioactive iodine can be passed on to children through the mother's milk, the children's thyroids may have been at risk. However, thyroid activity in nursing children was not measured directly in the AAL study.

Additionally, there was a possibility that a 30-year-old Arctic Village Athabaskan Indian woman may have been pregnant at the time of her participation in the I-131 studies. The Committee's report suggests that if the participant was pregnant at the time, she received a single dose of 50 microcuries in October 1955, the dose to the embryo is estimated to be 0.05 rad based on exposure to the embryo/fetus from accumulation of radioiodine in the mother's urinary bladder. Given the uncertainty, it is also unknown when this exposure might have occurred concerning gestational age. However, because of the small dose, the risk of developmental abnormalities and other untoward pregnancy outcomes is small.

These inclusions highlight significant ethical concerns, particularly by today's standards, regarding the protection of vulnerable populations in research studies.

Participants were administered I-131 in capsule form to measure thyroid activity. The dosage varied, but the standard procedure involved administering approximately 50 microcuries of I-131. While 50 microcuries was the standard dose for thyroid scans in the mid-1950s, today the standard dose is between 1–5 microcuries. Some subjects received multiple doses at intervals of one to six months. Measurements of thyroid uptake of radioiodide were taken at various times after administration, along with urinary and salivary excretion rates and blood levels of I-131.

The AAL study's documentation does not extensively detail the follow-up procedures for participants after the administration of I-131. The primary focus was on the immediate measurement of thyroid activity following I-131 administration rather than long-term health monitoring. However, the lack of systematic medical follow-up to determine the

---

[57] Rodahl, K. and Bang, G. (1957). Thyroid Activity in Men Exposed to Cold. Artic Aeromedical laboratory, Ladd Air Force Base, Alaska, Technical Report, 57–36.

long-term effects of I-131 administration on participants has been noted as a limitation of the study.

The procedures for obtaining informed consent from the study participants in the AAL experiments were not consistent with modern standards. According to the available reports, detailed informed consent processes, as understood today, were not followed. In the case of Alaska Natives, it appears that consent was obtained through discussions with village elders rather than directly with each participant. There is no evidence of written consent forms being used. For military personnel, the process involved briefing by the researchers and an opportunity to volunteer, but detailed documentation of informed consent procedures, including the explanation of risks and benefits, is lacking.

The AAL's thyroid function study found no significant differences in the absorption or elimination of radioactive tracers between Native and white participants nor did it find any evidence that cold exposure increased thyroid activity. The study, conducted by Rodahl and Bang (see footnote 32), determined that there were no differences based on race in how I-131 and its protein-bound form were absorbed or eliminated, and it also found no consistent changes across different seasons. The study observed that the higher absorption of I-131 among inland Inupiat Eskimos and Athabascan Indians from mountainous regions was due to a lack of iodine in their diets rather than cold exposure. Additionally, military subjects undergoing winter field exercises showed no signs of increased thyroid stimulation. The researchers concluded that the thyroid gland does not significantly contribute to the human body's adaptation to cold Arctic conditions.

Acceptable Radiation Exposure

On July 25, 1975, the FDA established for the first time limits on radiation to adult human volunteer research subjects.[58] The amount of radioactive

---

[58] U.S. Department of Health and Human Services Food and Drug Administration Center for Drug Evaluation and Research Center for Biologics Evaluation and Research August 2010 Clinical/Medical OMB Control No. 0910-0053, CFR – Code of Federal Regulations Title 21.

material administered to human research subjects during a research project intended to obtain basic information regarding the metabolism (e.g., kinetics, distribution, and localization) of a radioactively labeled drug should be the smallest radiation dose that can be administered without jeopardizing the benefits to be obtained from the study. The limit for the thyroid gland is 5 rad as a single dose and 15 rad as a cumulative dose from several studies conducted within one year. For children (research subjects under 18 years of age), limits are 10% of adult limits. Thyroid doses below these levels are generally recognized as safe (Department of Health and Human Services, 1990; Mossman, 1992). The major drawback of I-131 is the relatively high radiation dose received by the thyroid. Assuming an uptake of 25% of the administered radiation activity, the thyroid receives a dose of approximately 1.3 rad. per microcurie of administered radioactivity. In these experiments, the patients were exposed to 65 rads per dose.

Today's guidelines for radiation exposure, especially for research subjects, are significantly stricter than those during the 1950s. The contemporary understanding emphasizes a "no-threshold" philosophy, acknowledging that any radiation dose carries potential risk. This perspective marks a significant departure from the threshold-based approach prevalent during the AAL study period.

The AAL study's employment of I-131 and the subsequent assessment of its health impacts illustrate the evolution of our understanding of radiation safety and ethical considerations in medical research. While the study was conducted according to the guidelines and knowledge available at the time, current standards would likely preclude such an approach.

The ethical lapses found in this experiment are numerous and include the following:

1. **Informed Consent**: One of the most significant ethical lapses was the apparent lack of informed consent from the subjects. The study involved administering radioactive iodine (I-131) to Alaska Natives and military personnel without adequately explaining the nature of the experiments, the potential risks involved, or the fact that the research was non-therapeutic. Subjects were not always fully informed about the use of a radioactive substance and its potential health implications.

This lack of informed consent violates the principle of respect for persons, which requires that individuals are treated as autonomous agents and that those with diminished autonomy are entitled to protection.

2. **Use of Vulnerable Populations**: The study disproportionately involved Alaska Natives, including potentially pregnant or lactating women, without special considerations for their vulnerability. The selection of these populations raises concerns about exploitation and the principle of justice, which demands equitable distribution of research benefits and burdens. The use of vulnerable populations without adequate protections or consideration of their specific needs and without ensuring their understanding of the research represents a significant ethical lapse.

3. **Lack of Follow-up Care**: There was no systematic follow-up care or monitoring for participants to identify potential long-term effects of exposure to radioactive iodine. This neglect disregards the principle of beneficence, which obligates researchers to maximize benefits and minimize harm to research subjects.

4. **Potential Coercion**: The recruitment methods and the context in which consent was obtained may have involved elements of coercion or undue influence, particularly given the hierarchical nature of military environments and the socio-economic conditions of the Alaska Native populations. This compromises the voluntariness of the consent.

5. **Lack of Transparency and Accountability**: The study's design, risks, and results were not transparently communicated to the subjects or the wider community, undermining the trust in and the integrity of the research process.

6. **Ethical Review and Oversight**: The experiments were conducted in a period when formal ethical review boards (Institutional Review Boards or IRBs) were not yet a standard requirement for research involving human subjects. However, the lack of any apparent independent ethical review of the study's protocol and its risks versus benefits represents a lapse in ensuring the ethical conduct of the research.

The AAL's thyroid function study conducted in the 1950s, which involved the administration of radioactive iodine (I-131) to Alaska Natives and military personnel, stands as a significant historical example of the ethical complexities and challenges inherent in human subject research. This study aimed to understand the role of the thyroid in acclimatization to cold environments, yet it unfolded within a framework that, by today's standards, inadequately protected the rights and welfare of its participants.

The ethical lapses identified in the conduct of the AAL experiments — such as the lack of informed consent, the use of vulnerable populations without adequate protections, the absence of follow-up care, potential coercion in participant recruitment, and the lack of transparency and accountability — highlight the critical importance of ethical oversight in research. These lapses underscore the necessity of adhering to ethical principles that respect the autonomy, dignity, and rights of research participants.

The aftermath of the AAL study and similar research endeavors of its time contributed to a profound shift in the ethical landscape of human subject research. They catalyzed the development and implementation of ethical guidelines, such as the Belmont Report, and the establishment of IRBs to ensure that research involving human participants is conducted in a manner that prioritizes their safety, dignity, and rights above the pursuit of scientific knowledge.

Furthermore, the AAL experiments serve as a reminder of the ongoing need for vigilance, education, and ethical sensitivity in research practices. They emphasize the importance of informed consent as a fundamental tenet of ethical research, the necessity of equitable treatment of all research participants, and the imperative of providing adequate care and follow-up for those who choose to participate in research.

The AAL thyroid function study is a pivotal chapter in the history of research ethics, serving both as a cautionary tale and as a catalyst for positive change. It reminds us of the paramount importance of ethical considerations in the conduct of research and the responsibility of the scientific community to protect the welfare of human subjects. As we move forward, it is crucial that the lessons learned from the AAL experiments and similar studies inform current and future research practices, ensuring that the pursuit of scientific knowledge is always balanced with respect for human rights and dignity.

Conclusion

The exploration of the Fernald State School, Cincinnati Radiation, Holmesburg Prison, and Alaskan Iodine-131 experiments within this chapter illuminates a dark era in medical research, where the quest for scientific advancement often eclipsed the fundamental rights and well-being of individuals. These studies, characterized by the use of radioactive substances on unwitting and vulnerable populations, highlight critical lapses in ethical judgment and a profound disregard for human dignity. As we conclude this examination, it is crucial to recognize these historical missteps not merely as relics of the past but as enduring lessons on the importance of ethical integrity in research. The legacy of these experiments compels us to uphold the highest standards of consent, transparency, and respect for all research subjects, ensuring that the horrors of yesterday do not become the failures of tomorrow. In moving forward, let the stories of those affected by these experiments reinforce our collective resolve to place human rights at the forefront of scientific inquiry, safeguarding against the repetition of such ethical transgressions.

Further Reading

For those interested in delving deeper into the ethical, historical, and medical aspects of the Fernald State School experiments, the Cincinnati Radiation Experiments, the Holmesburg Prison experiments, and the Alaskan Iodine-131 study, the following reading list offers a comprehensive starting point:

1. **"The Plutonium Files: America's Secret Medical Experiments in the Cold War" by Eileen Welsome**
   - This Pulitzer Prize-winning book provides an in-depth look at the U.S. government's secret medical experiments during the Cold War, including the use of radioactive substances on unwitting subjects.

2. **"Acres of Skin: Human Experiments at Holmesburg Prison" by Allen M. Hornblum**
   - Hornblum's book focuses on the unethical medical experiments conducted on inmates at Holmesburg Prison, offering a detailed account of the studies and their implications.

3. **"Against Their Will: The Secret History of Medical Experimentation on Children in Cold War America" by Allen M. Hornblum, Judith L. Newman, and Gregory J. Dober**
   - This work explores the history of medical experimentation on children, including those at the Fernald State School, highlighting the ethical breaches and the impact on the subjects.

4. **"Undue Risk: Secret State Experiments on Humans" by Jonathan D. Moreno**
   - Moreno's book examines the history of human experimentation by the U.S. government, including radiation studies and other secret projects, providing a critical analysis of the ethical considerations.

5. **"The Treatment: The Story of Those Who Died in the Cincinnati Radiation Tests" by Martha Stephens**
   - Focusing on the Cincinnati Radiation Experiments, Stephens' book offers a poignant look at the lives affected by these tests and the ethical questions they raise.

6. **"Ethical and Legal Issues in Human Experimentation" by Bernard Barber (Editor)**
   - This collection of essays addresses the broader ethical and legal challenges of human experimentation, providing context for understanding the specific cases mentioned.

7. **"Journey into Darkness: The Unauthorized History of Secret Medical Experiments in the Cold War" by Gordon Thomas**
   - Thomas' book delves into the covert world of Cold War medical experiments, including those involving radiation, offering insights into the motivations and outcomes.

8. **"In the Name of Science: A History of Secret Programs, Medical Research, and Human Experimentation" by Andrew Goliszek**
   - This work provides an overview of secret medical research and human experimentation, including discussions on the ethical implications and historical context.

9. **"Medical Apartheid: The Dark History of Medical Experimentation on Black Americans from Colonial Times to the Present" by Harriet A. Washington**

- While focusing on the African American experience, Washington's book offers valuable insights into the broader history of medical experimentation, including studies like those at Holmesburg Prison.

These books provide a foundation for understanding the complex ethical, historical, and medical dimensions of the experiments conducted at Fernald State School, Cincinnati, Holmesburg Prison, and Alaska, offering readers a pathway to further explore the implications and lessons of these studies.

Chapter 6

The St. Louis Experiment

In the shadows of the Cold War, a chilling narrative unfolded in the streets of St. Louis, cloaked in the secrecy of military endeavors and the guise of public safety. Operation Large Area Coverage, a covert program orchestrated by the U.S. Army Chemical Corps, saw the city's most impoverished neighborhoods become the testing ground for a hazardous experiment. With the release of zinc cadmium sulfide — a compound whose health implications remain a subject of disconcerting ambiguity — the military ventured into a realm of ethical obscurity. The program's architects, ensconced in the silence of classified operations, eschewed transparency, leaving an unwitting public vulnerable to the caprices of a toxic plume. This chapter delves into the enigmatic depths of an operation that epitomized the era's flagrant disregard for individual rights, unraveling a tapestry of subterfuge and the ineradicable scars it left upon the American psyche.

The experiments conducted in St. Louis, Missouri, in the 1950s and 1960s, were part of a series of secretive tests aimed at understanding how to prepare for potential biological or chemical attacks.[1] These military tests were named "Operation — Large Area Coverage" or LAC.

The St. Louis Experiment, conducted in the mid-20th century, was part of a broader series of tests by the United States government aimed

---

[1] National Research Council (US) (1997). *Toxicologic Assessment of the Army's Zinc Cadmium Sulfide Dispersion Tests*. National Academies Press (US). pp. Appendix A: Zinc Cadmium Sulfide Dispersion Tests.

at understanding the potential for chemical and biological warfare defense. This set of experiments focused on analyzing the urban dispersal of small particles. The primary objective was to simulate a biological or chemical weapons attack. Specifically, the experiment aimed to simulate how biological or chemical weapons, if deployed by enemy forces, would spread through the air across densely populated areas. This knowledge was deemed crucial for developing effective countermeasures and evacuation plans to protect the civilian population in the event of such attacks.

Zinc cadmium sulfide, a fine powder, was used in these experiments While not a biological weapon, it served as a tracer in simulations to study the spread of biological weapons in different settings. This inorganic compound, made up of zinc, cadmium, and sulfur, emits a bright yellow or green glow under ultraviolet light, facilitating its easy detection. It was selected for these experiments due to its ability to be easily tracked either visually or through special detection devices. At the time of the experiments, the use of zinc cadmium sulfide was not considered a health risk. The compound was chosen precisely because it was thought to pose no harm, allowing researchers to focus on the dispersal patterns without concern for immediate public health implications. However, this assessment of harmlessness was based on the limited toxicological understanding of the time and did not account for the long-term effects of cadmium exposure, which would later be recognized for its potential to cause serious health issues, including kidney damage, bone fractures, and cancer.

This assumption of safety did not justify the lack of transparency with the subjects regarding their involvement and the potential health implications. The subsequent public discovery of the experiment highlighted severe breaches of trust and ethical standards, particularly concerning the rights and welfare of the participants.

The experimental protocol called for dispersing zinc cadmium sulfide from various platforms. Motorized blowers were installed in airplanes, on towers, and the rooftops of buildings, and from moving station wagons, to mimic the dispersal mechanisms that might be used in warfare.

Samples were collected at various distances from the release points to analyze the geographic range, dispersal patterns, and concentration levels of

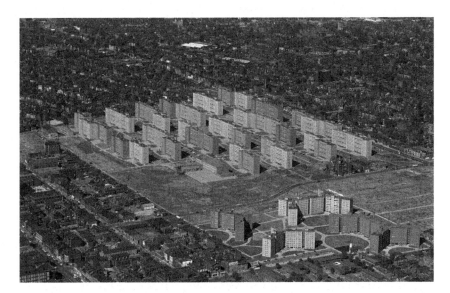

Figure 1. The Pruit-Igoe Housing Complex, St. Louis Missouri.

Source: Wiki Commons.

the particles in the air.[2] This data was intended to provide insights into how a biological or chemical agent might behave under similar conditions.

The Pruitt-Igoe housing complex was one of the primary sites for these experiments (Figure 1). This complex was one of the largest housing projects in the world. Located on the north side of St. Louis, it consisted of 33 eleven-story high-rise buildings on 57 acres.[3] At its highest occupancy, it held 10,000 people. The project was designed for the working poor, and although it was legally integrated, it was almost exclusively occupied by African Americans. The government's selection of Pruitt-Igoe and similar locations highlighted a disturbing trend of conducting potentially hazardous tests in areas inhabited by minority and poor populations.

Research into the tests, including investigations by journalists and scholars, has highlighted the potential for racial and socio-economic biases in the selection of test sites. Critics argue that the choice of

[2] Novick, L.F. and Marr, J.S. (2003). *Public Health Issues Disaster Preparedness: Focus on Bioterrorism*, (Google Books), Jones & Bartlett Publishers. p. 89.

[3] Bristol, K. (1991). The Pruitt–Igoe Myth. *Journal of Architectural Education*. 44(3): 163–171. doi: 10.1080/10464883.1991.11102687.

locations reflects a pattern of exploiting vulnerable populations for scientific and military research, a pattern seen in other instances of environmental and experimental injustice.[4]

The experiment was conceived and designed by a team within the U.S. Army and the Atomic Energy Commission, to understand the dispersion of florescent particles as a proxy for biological and chemical warfare agents. The architect of this program is unknown and even the names of the team members remain nameless due to the secret nature of the tests. This team comprised military strategists, scientists, and experts in chemical and biological warfare, who together identified the objectives and methodologies that would be employed in the experiment. Their collaboration ensured that the experiment's design was grounded in the latest scientific knowledge and aligned with national defense priorities.

The responsibility for carrying out the experiment fell to a combination of military personnel, government contractors, and research institutions. The U.S. Army, particularly its Chemical Corps, played a pivotal role in the operational aspects of the experiment, overseeing the dispersal of zinc cadmium sulfide and the subsequent data collection.[5] Contractors and research institutions, including Stanford University and the Ralph Parsons Company, were enlisted for their technical expertise and resources, contributing to the execution of the dispersion tests and the analysis of environmental and health data.

The experiment was supported by a robust structure of funding and authorization that spanned several branches of the U.S. government. Financial backing primarily came from the U.S. Army's budget, allocated for research and development in national defense, with additional support from the Atomic Energy Commission, reflecting the experiment's significance to both military preparedness and atomic energy research. Authorization for the experiment was secured through a series of approvals at various levels of the government, ensuring that it was conducted

---

[4] https://www.weforum.org/agenda/2020/07/what-is-environmental-racism-pollution-covid-systemic/ (Accessed 2/6/24).

[5] Guillemin, J. (2005). *Biological Weapons: From the Invention of State-Sponsored Programs to Contemporary Bioterrorism*, (Internet Archive), Columbia University Press. p. 108.

within the legal and ethical frameworks of the time. This process involved not only the military and the Atomic Energy Commission but also local government entities in the areas where the tests were conducted, who were often kept in the dark about the full implications of the experiments.

The areas selected for the dispersion tests were primarily urban environments across the United States and Canada, with a notable emphasis on regions that housed poor and minority populations. The selection process was influenced by a set of criteria that included population density, geographical features, and the logistical feasibility of conducting the dispersion tests without arousing public suspicion. The Pruitt-Igoe housing complex in St. Louis, predominantly inhabited by African American residents, emerged as a focal point for the experiments due to its high-density living conditions and the ease with which the area could be monitored and studied.

These experiments egregiously violated several core ethical principles, which are now foundational to the field of bioethics. The principle of autonomy was compromised as individuals in the St. Louis area were not informed about the experiments nor was their consent sought, stripping them of their right to make informed decisions about their participation. This directly undermines the individual's freedom and agency, a right that is enshrined in the Nuremberg Code and later, the Declaration of Helsinki, which emphasizes the importance of voluntary, informed consent in all human subject research. The principle of non-maleficence, which obliges researchers to avoid causing harm, was also violated. Although the government and the Army believed that zinc cadmium sulfide was harmless, the long-term exposure and health implications were not fully understood, and the lack of post-experiment follow-up disregarded the need to prevent harm to the participants.[6]

Beneficence, the duty to promote good and act in the best interest of the participants and society, was ignored as the experiments were designed

---

[6]National Research Council (US) Committee on Toxicology. (1997). *Toxicologic Assessment of the Army's Zinc Cadmium Sulfide Dispersion Tests: Answers to Commonly Asked Questions.* Washington (DC): National Academies Press (US). Toxicologic Assessment of the Army's Zinc Cadmium Sulfide Dispersion Tests: Answers to Commonly Asked Questions. Available from: https://www.ncbi.nlm.nih.gov/books/NBK233549/.

to benefit the U.S. military's chemical and biological weapons program, not the individuals exposed or the community at large. Lastly, the principle of justice was not upheld, as the experiments disproportionately targeted poor and African American communities, perpetuating a legacy of exploitation and research abuse against marginalized groups. This is a stark violation of the justice principle, which demands equitable distribution of both the burdens and benefits of research. Current ethical guidelines, including those outlined by the AMA Code of Medical Ethics, seek to prevent such abuses by emphasizing the role of informed consent, the necessity of risk minimization, and the importance of equitable selection of research subjects to ensure that the wrongs of the past are not repeated.

The failure to obtain informed consent from the residents of Pruitt-Igoe and other test sites not only compromised the ethical integrity of the experiment but also contributed to a legacy of mistrust toward government and scientific institutions within these communities.

This decision-making process failed to consider the potential health risks associated with exposure to zinc cadmium sulfide, however minimal they were believed to be at the time. Therefore, no systematic health monitoring of the exposed populations was conducted. As a result, there was a lack of real-time health surveillance that could have provided immediate data on the impact of exposure.

In the years following the public disclosure of the experiment, concerns raised by affected communities prompted retrospective analyses and health studies.[7] The US Occupational Safety and Health Administration states that "cadmium and its compounds are highly toxic and exposure to this metal is known to cause cancer and targets the body's cardiovascular, renal, gastrointestinal, neurological, reproductive, and respiratory systems." While this is true of pure cadmium metal, the health effects of this compound of cadmium were unclear. Some evidence was proposed suggesting that zinc cadmium sulfide caused adverse health effects in the study population.[8]

---

[7] https://www.cbsnews.com/news/secret-cold-war-tests-in-st-louis-cause-worry/ (Accessed 2/6/24).

[8] LeBaron, W. (1998). *America's Nuclear Legacy*, (Google Books), Nova Publishers. p. 83–84.

This raised concerns among the public and especially among those who were exposed. In response to these concerns, Congress tasked the National Research Council (NRC), an independent and non-partisan body that addresses science and technology issues, with investigating whether the Army's zinc cadmium sulfide tests had led to any harmful health effects. To carry out this investigation, the NRC established a subcommittee within its Committee on Toxicology, which is part of the Board on Environmental Studies and Toxicology.[9] This subcommittee was responsible for conducting a thorough study.

The claims of public harm were challenged due to lack of evidence. By the time the investigations began, the buildings had been leveled and the residents dispersed, which made collecting health or environmental information difficult. Further, it was impossible to directly link health outcomes to the experiment due to the lack of baseline health data of the populace and the presence of multiple environmental and lifestyle factors that could influence health.

To evaluate the potential risk to individuals exposed to zinc cadmium sulfide, a specialized subcommittee of the NRC focused on exposure to cadmium, the compound's most hazardous component. The subcommittee determined that the levels of cadmium present in the zinc cadmium sulfide dispersed during the Army's tests were significantly lower than the thresholds known to cause toxic effects. Specifically, in St. Louis, the area with the highest exposure, the maximum estimated airborne cadmium exposure (24.4 micrograms) was comparable to the amount of cadmium that urban residents might typically breathe in over a period ranging from 1–8 months.[10] The U.S. NRC concluded that "After an exhaustive, independent review requested by Congress, we have found no evidence that exposure to zinc cadmium sulfide at these levels could cause people to become

---

[9] National Research Council (US). (1997). *Toxicologic Assessment of the Army's Zinc Cadmium Sulfide Dispersion Tests*. National Academies Press (US). pp. Appendix A: Zinc Cadmium Sulfide Dispersion Tests.

[10] National Research Council (US) Committee on Toxicology. (1997). *Toxicologic Assessment of the Army's Zinc Cadmium Sulfide Dispersion Tests: Answers to Commonly Asked Questions*. Washington (DC): National Academies Press (US). Available from: https://www.ncbi.nlm.nih.gov/books/NBK233549/.

sick."[11] However, there is no information available on the potential toxicity of the particles in the lung. It is also not known whether ZnCdS can be broken down by pulmonary macrophages into more soluble and toxic forms of cadmium.[12]

The St. Louis Experiment remained classified and unknown to the public for several decades, with its existence and details only coming to light in the early 1990s. This delay in disclosure meant that an entire generation of residents lived without knowledge of the potential exposure to hazardous substances.

The revelation of the experiment had profound implications for public perception and trust in government and scientific research. Discovering that the government had conducted secret tests, using potentially hazardous substances on unsuspecting citizens, particularly in disadvantaged and minority communities, led to widespread outrage and skepticism with one critic accusing the US Army of "using the country as an experimental laboratory."[13] This breach of trust has had lasting effects, contributing to a cautious or even distrustful view of government-sponsored health and environmental research.[14]

The exposure of the St. Louis Experiment prompted significant legal and regulatory changes aimed at safeguarding the ethical treatment of research subjects. This period saw the reinforcement of the Common Rule and the publication of the Belmont Report, which established key ethical principles in research involving human subjects. Institutional Review Boards (IRBs) were strengthened to ensure rigorous ethical review of research proposals, emphasizing the necessity of informed consent,

---

[11] Leary, W.E. (May 15, 1997). Secret Army Chemical Tests Did Not Harm Health. Report Says, *The New York Times* (Accessed 13/11/08).

[12] National Research Council (US) Subcommittee on Zinc Cadmium Sulfide. (1997). *Toxicologic Assessment of the Army's Zinc Cadmium Sulfide Dispersion Tests.* Washington (DC): National Academies Press (US). 3, Toxicity and Related Data on Zinc Cadmium Sulfide. Available from: https://www.ncbi.nlm.nih.gov/books/NBK233497/.

[13] Moreno, J.D. (2001). *Undue Risk: Secret State Experiments on Humans*, Routledge. p. 235.

[14] https://www.nbcnews.com/news/us-news/-experimented-victims-secret-cold-war-testing-st-louis-demand-compensa-rcna117149 (Accessed 2/6/24).

transparency, and accountability. These developments have profoundly influenced the conduct of human subject research, embedding respect for individual rights and welfare at the core of scientific inquiry and ensuring that the ethical oversights of the past are not repeated.

Despite the public revelation of the details of this experiment, there has been limited progress in providing compensation to affected subjects or their families (see footnote 12). Efforts to secure compensation have been hampered by challenges in linking health issues directly to the experiment and legal obstacles.[15]

In a similar vein, despite the acknowledgment of the people and institutions responsible for this experiment, there is scant evidence of sanctions or legal repercussions for those who designed and implemented the experiment. Despite the ethical violations identified, specific disciplinary actions against the individuals involved have not been widely reported. Instead, the experiment has prompted significant reforms in research ethics, leading to stronger protections for research participants. While these reforms do not directly redress the grievances of those affected by the experiment, they serve to prevent similar ethical lapses in future research endeavors.

The St. Louis Experiment has had a profound impact on ethical research practices, serving as a pivotal case study in the evolution of research ethics. The experiment's lack of informed consent and its selection of vulnerable populations without their knowledge highlighted significant ethical shortcomings, leading to a reevaluation of how research is conducted, especially regarding human subjects. The public outcry and subsequent scrutiny catalyzed the strengthening of ethical guidelines.

The ethical landscape of modern research, particularly in the domains of digital and genetic data collection, presents an echo of the same questions of consent and human dignity that the St. Louis Experiments laid bare. Today, the field of genetic research, with its power to unlock the most intimate personal data, amplifies the essentiality of informed

---

[15] https://www.nbcnews.com/news/us-news/-experimented-victims-secret-cold-war-testing-st-louis-demand-compensa-rcna117149 (Accessed 6/25/24).

consent, a subject of much legal and moral discussion.[16,17] As we navigate the complexities of genomic studies, the right to privacy, and the line between personal autonomy and the public good, the St. Louis case study becomes a cautionary touchstone. It reminds us that the seductive pull of progress, whether in the name of public health or the next quantum leap in data science, must never outstrip our collective ethical vigilance. The case of the St. Louis Experiments, while a chronicle of a bygone era, is a mirror to our own, reflecting the invariable human need to balance the hunger for knowledge with the inalienable right to self-determination and respect for individual agency.[18,19]

Reflecting on the lessons learned from the St. Louis Experiment, it's clear that ethical vigilance is paramount in safeguarding the dignity and welfare of research subjects. The experiment underscores the importance of ethical oversight mechanisms, such as IRBs, in ensuring research is conducted with the highest ethical standards. Moreover, it highlights the need for ongoing education and awareness among researchers and the public about the ethical dimensions of scientific inquiry.

The ongoing implications for human subject research are significant. The St. Louis Experiment serves as a reminder of the potential consequences when ethical considerations are sidelined. It emphasizes that the pursuit of scientific knowledge must always be balanced with respect for individual rights and well-being.

As research continues to evolve, particularly in areas involving new technologies and methodologies, the lessons from the St. Louis Experiment remain relevant, guiding the ethical conduct of research to ensure that past mistakes are not repeated.

---

[16] Lee, S.S. (2021). The ethics of consent in a shifting genomic ecosystem. *Annu Rev Biomed Data Sci.* 4:145–164. doi: 10.1146/annurev-biodatasci-030221-125715.

[17] Ethical Challenges in Obtaining Informed Consent for Genetic/Genomic Research https://elsihub.org/collection/ethical-challenges-obtaining-informed-consent-genetic genomic-research (Accessed 2/20/24).

[18] https://www.acog.org/clinical/clinical-guidance/committee-opinion/articles/2008/06/ ethical-issues-in-genetic-testing (Accessed 2/20/24).

[19] Mezinska, S., Gallagher, L. and Verbrugge, M. *et al.* (2021). Ethical issues in genomics research on neurodevelopmental disorders: a critical interpretive review. *Hum Genomics.* **15**, article 16. https://doi.org/10.1186/s40246-021-00317-4.

Chapter 7

MK-Ultra Program

During the early stages of the Cold War, the human mind emerged as a covert battlefront where both sides developed new methods of mass persuasion and individual interrogation, seeking any possible advantage that could be leveraged in this global standoff.

Between 1950 and 1962, the CIA spearheaded an extensive and clandestine research initiative aimed at unlocking the secrets of human consciousness. It was called MK-Ultra. This initiative, akin to a psychological Manhattan Project, saw its annual budget for psychological research and operations soar to a billion dollars at its height.[1]

Started in 1951 as Project Artichoke, it was renamed MK-Ultra in 1953, and its precursor represented the United States government's foray into the manipulation of human consciousness and its attempts at mastering mind control. These efforts were driven by a mix of fear and ambition, aiming to develop abilities for improved interrogation, behavior modification, and psychological warfare that could counter perceived threats from adversaries on the global stage.

For instance, the Soviet Union's use of psychiatric hospitals to suppress dissent and enforce ideological conformity, along with sophisticated methods of interrogation and indoctrination possibly involving drugs and psychological pressure, contributed to fears in the West about mind control. Similarly, information about Chinese mind control programs was gleaned

---

[1] Simpson, C. (1994). *Science of Coercion: Communication Research & Psychological Warfare 1945–1960.* New York: Oxford University Press.

from the treatment of American prisoners of war during the Korean War, with reports that returning American POWs had been "brainwashed" while in captivity, further fueling the urgency to develop countermeasures. These historical and geopolitical factors set the stage for the United States to embark on its secretive experiments aimed at exploring the possibilities of controlling human behavior through the manipulation of mental states and altering brain functions, leading to the establishment of MK-Ultra and Project ARTICHOKE. The significance of these programs extends far beyond their historical context, touching on core issues of medical ethics, the relationship between science and state power, and the evolution of ethical standards in medical and psychological research.

The significance of MK-Ultra extends far beyond its historical context, touching on core issues of medical ethics and the relationship between science and state power. This program conducted experiments that ranged from the administration of psychoactive drugs, including Lysergic Acid Diethylamide (LSD), to hypnosis, sensory deprivation, and a host of other techniques, often on unwitting subjects. The ethical breaches committed in the name of national security — such as the lack of informed consent, the deliberate deception of research subjects, and the exposure of participants to potentially harmful substances without regard for their well-being — raise profound questions about the limits of scientific inquiry and the responsibilities of researchers.

Discussing MK-Ultra is crucial not only for understanding a dark chapter in American history but also for appreciating the evolution of ethical standards in medical and psychological research. These programs prompted significant scrutiny and criticism once they were brought to light, contributing to the establishment of more rigorous ethical guidelines for research involving human subjects. Today, the legacy of MK-Ultra and Project ARTICHOKE serves as a cautionary tale about the potential for abuse when scientific research is conducted without stringent ethical oversight and transparency.

This chapter aims to provide an overview of the MK-Ultra and Project ARTICHOKE programs, examining the ethical breaches they entailed and their lasting impact on the field of medical research. By exploring this troubling yet pivotal story, we can gain insights into the importance of ethical vigilance and the need to balance scientific curiosity with the imperative to protect the rights and dignity of individuals.

Historical Context and Justification

The Cold War era, marked by intense rivalry between the United States and the Soviet Union, was a period of geopolitical tension and ideological conflict that lasted from the end of World War II in 1945 until the dissolution of the Soviet Union in 1991. This era was characterized by mutual distrust, the threat of nuclear warfare, and a race for technological and ideological superiority. Within this context, both superpowers engaged in extensive espionage and sought any possible advantage that could be leveraged in this global standoff.

Amid these tensions, the U.S. government's interest in developing mind control emerged not merely as a speculative endeavor but as a perceived necessity. The initial motivations for projects like MK-Ultra and Project ARTICHOKE were rooted in the fear of falling behind the Soviet Union and the People's Republic of China, which were rumored to be making significant advances in psychological warfare.[2]

For example, the Soviet Union was reported to use psychiatric hospitals as a means of suppressing dissent and enforcing ideological conformity. While more widely recognized during the later Cold War years, concerns about such practices were already emerging in the 1950s. The use of psychiatric evaluation and treatment as tools of political control contributed to fears in the West about mind control.

The first instance of apparent mind control noticed in the West was the 1949 trial of Józef Cardinal Mindszenty (Figure 1). The communist government charged the Roman Catholic Primate of Hungary with treason. During the trial, Cardinal Mindszenty appeared confused, spoke in a flat, unemotional voice, and admitted to crimes there was clear evidence he hadn't committed.[3] Defectors and intelligence reports suggested that the

---

[2] Williams, C. (2020) Public psychology and the Cold War brainwashing scare. *Hist Philos Psychol.* 21(1):21–30.

[3] Streatfield, D. (2007) *Brainwash: The Secret History of Mind Control.* New York, NY: Thomas Dunne Books.

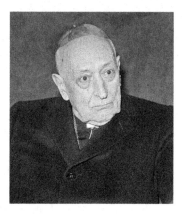

Figure 1. Józef Cardial Mindszensky, 1974.
Source: Image Wiki Commons.

Soviets had developed sophisticated methods of interrogation and indoctrination, possibly involving drugs, psychological pressure, and brainwashing, especially through the application of their "reflexive control" techniques.[4] Reflexive control refers to the technique of presenting specially crafted information to someone, whether a collaborator or adversary, in such a way that it leads them to voluntarily decide what the person initiating this action wants them to. These methods were believed to be part of a broader strategy to ensure loyalty and control over individuals, particularly those with access to sensitive information.

Information about Chinese mind control was gleaned from the treatment of the American prisoners of war during the Korean War.[5] The Chinese government's use of thought reform and re-education camps was another source of concern. These camps aimed to "re-educate" political dissidents, counter-revolutionaries, and others through a combination of ideological indoctrination, self-criticism sessions, and sometimes harsh treatments. The goal was to align individuals' beliefs and behaviors with Communist Party doctrine.

---

[4] https://archive.org/details/soviettheoryofre00chot/mode/1up (Accessed 2/7/24).
[5] Brain-washing in Red China: The calculated destruction of men's minds Hardcover — January 1, 1951 by Edward Hunter. Vanguard Press; 1st edition (January 1, 1951), pp. 295–297.

Edward Hunter, a journalist and former OSS officer, was the pioneer in raising awareness with his headline, "Brain-washing Tactics Force Chinese Into Ranks of Communist Party," in the *Miami Daily News* in September 1950. Through his writings, both in articles and subsequently in a book,[6] Hunter detailed how the Red Army, under Mao Zedong, employed ancient methods to transform the populace of China into obedient followers of Communism. Hunter introduced the term "brainwashing," directly translating the Mandarin xi-nao, meaning to wash (xi) and brain (nao), highlighting its potential perilous uses.[7]

Reports that returning American POWs of the Korean War had been "brainwashed" while in captivity led to significant concern in the United States. For example, 5,000 of the 7,200 US POWs either petitioned the US government to end the war or signed confessions of their alleged crimes. Other POWs were filmed making anti-American statements or confessing to war crimes while in captivity, actions that were attributed to Chinese indoctrination and mind control programs.[8] The final blow came at the end of the Korean War, when 23 US Army soldiers, who were prisoners of war in Korea, chose to live in China instead of returning home.[9] While the US military denied all the charges leveled at it by the POWs, they couldn't explain what had made them make these statements. The only explanation, in their minds, was brainwashing.

In fact, people who took time to study the POWs found a far simpler explanation for their behavior, they were tortured.

Nevertheless, this fear of brainwashing was so intense that all returning American POWs were treated as collaborators, potential spies, and

---

[6] Brainwashing: Its History; Use by Totalitarian Communist Regimes; and Stories of American and British Soldiers and Captives Who Defied It, Edward Hunter, Pantianos Classics (January 1, 1956), pp. 93–94.

[7] https://www.smithsonianmag.com/history/true-story-brainwashing-and-how-it-shaped-america-180963400/ (Accessed 2/22/24).

[8] Carruthers, S.L. (2009). *Cold War captives: Imprisonment, escape, and brainwashing*. Berkely: University of California Press.

[9] Lautz, T. (2022). Clarence Adams and Morris Wills: Searching for utopia. *Americans in China: Encounters with the People's Republic*, New York, p. 41–C2.P84. Online edn, Oxford Academic, 20 Jan. 2022, https://doi.org/10.1093/oso/9780197512838.003.0003 (Accessed 2/9/2024).

threats to national security. These POWs, after suffering the privations of a North Korean POW camp for years, often underwent prolonged and aggressive interrogations by the American Military to try to understand why American Soldiers wouldn't want to return home.[10] US Military authorities reasoned that if the Chinese could convince some soldiers to stay behind, it was possible they could convince others to carry out espionage missions upon their return to the United States.

These reports of "brainwashing" used on U.S. prisoners of war during the Korean War further fueled the urgency to develop methods for mind control, interrogation, and indoctrination that could counter these perceived threats and potentially be used to gain a strategic advantage over adversaries.[11]

MK-Ultra was officially sanctioned in 1953 by then-CIA Director Allen Dulles, and it became the most prominent of the CIA's mind control programs.[12] It aimed to explore the possibilities of controlling human behavior through the manipulation of mental states and altering brain functions. This included experiments with psychoactive drugs (most famously LSD), hypnosis, sensory deprivation, isolation, verbal and sexual abuse, and various forms of torture.

Project ARTICHOKE was initiated in 1951 with similar goals. It focused more specifically on interrogation methods and the possibility of creating an unwitting assassin or manipulating a subject to perform tasks against their will through mind control.[13]

The justification for these programs was deeply rooted in the Cold War's atmosphere of fear and the belief that the ends (protecting national security) justified the means (ethical breaches in experimentation). This rationale, however, led to significant ethical violations, including

---

[10] McKnight, B. (2014). *We Fight for Peace*, p.142. The Kent State University Press.

[11] Santucci, P.S. and Winokur, G. (1955). Brainwashing as a Factor in Psychiatric Illness: A Heuristic Approach. *AMA Arch NeurPsych.* 74(1):11–16. doi: 10.1001/archneurpsyc.1955. 02330130013003.

[12] https://www.scribd.com/document/75512716/Project-MKUltra-The-CIA-s-Program-of-Research-in-Behavioral-Modification (Accessed 2/7/24).

[13] chrome-extension://mhnlakgilnojmhinhkckjpncpbhabphi/pages/pdf/web/viewer.html?file=https%3A%2F%2Fnsarchive2.gwu.edu%2FNSAEBB%2FNSAEBB54%2Fst02.pdf (Accessed 2/7/24).

non-consensual experimentation on humans, which were later exposed and condemned.

The ethical implications of these programs are profound, raising questions about the limits of governmental authority in research, the necessity of informed consent, and the protection of individuals from harm. The revelations about MK-Ultra and Project ARTICHOKE contributed to a reevaluation of ethical standards in research, leading to the establishment of more stringent guidelines and oversight mechanisms, such as Institutional Review Boards (IRBs) in the United States.

Overview of MK-Ultra and Project ARTICHOKE

MK-Ultra was designed to develop mind control that could be used for interrogation purposes, to control individuals against their will, and to enhance the capabilities of U.S. intelligence operations.

One of the most surprising aspects of the MK-Ultra project is the sheer breadth and audacity of the experiments conducted under its auspices, including the use of LSD and other psychoactive drugs, in a quest for mind control. The program's experiments were not limited to willing participants or informed volunteers but extended to unsuspecting individuals, including U.S. citizens, who were subjected to drug administration and psychological manipulations without their consent. This included efforts to explore the potential of LSD to alter mental states and affect brain function, as well as investigations into hypnosis, sensory deprivation, and the potential for creating "Manchurian Candidates."[14]

Another surprising element is the involvement of reputable universities, hospitals, and research institutions, often without their knowledge of the project's true nature, funded through CIA front organizations to

---

[14] *The Manchurian Candidate* is a political thriller released in 1962. It explores the story of a group of American soldiers who are captured during the Korean War and brainwashed by Communists into becoming sleeper agents. The plot thickens when one of the soldiers, Raymond Shaw, returns to the United States as a decorated war hero, unknowingly programmed to assassinate a presidential candidate as part of a Communist conspiracy. The film delves into themes of power, manipulation, and the impact of mind control, culminating in a tense race against time to uncover the truth and prevent the assassination.

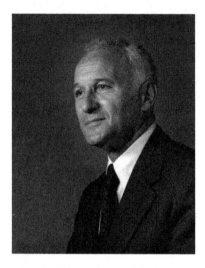

Figure 2.   Sidney Gottlieb, MD.
Source: Central Intelligence Agency Photo.

conduct experiments. The extent of collaboration with such institutions underscores the covert and deceptive methods employed by the CIA to advance the project's objectives.

Furthermore, the discovery that significant figures within the U.S. government and intelligence community authorized and supported such ethically dubious research reveals a troubling willingness to bypass moral and legal standards in the name of national security. The subsequent efforts to destroy evidence and cover up the program's existence, including the destruction of documents ordered by Sidney Gottlieb in 1973, add to the project's notorious legacy.

Project ARTICHOKE, initiated in 1951, was the precursor to MK-Ultra, initiated in 1951. It focused specifically on interrogation methods and the possibility of creating "Manchurian Candidates" — individuals who could be involuntarily programmed to perform assassinations or other missions without their knowledge or consent.

Sidney Gottlieb was an operative for the Central Intelligence Agency (CIA), where he played a central role in the MK-Ultra program (Figure 2). Gottlieb joined the CIA in 1951. By 1953, he was made the head of the Chemical Division of the Technical Services Staff (TSS), and shortly thereafter, he became the chief of MK-Ultra when it was officially sanctioned. Under his direction, MK-Ultra explored various methods for effective interrogation and mind control, including the use of LSD on unwitting subjects, sensory deprivation, and other psychological techniques.[15]

Gottlieb was deeply involved in the design and execution of MK-Ultra's experiments, both in the United States and abroad. Gottlieb was interested in understanding the effects of LSD on the human mind, particularly its potential use in interrogation and mind control. To this end, LSD was administered to unwitting subjects, including CIA employees, as part of the program's experiments.

His work included overseeing the administration of drugs to both volunteers and unwitting subjects to study its effects and potential utility in interrogation and mind control. He sponsored physicians such as Donald Ewen Cameron who we see in the following chapter. He was also involved in controversial psychiatric research, including non-consensual human experiments.[16]

A specific case of non-consensual drug administration involved a CIA employee named Frank Olson. Olsen was a bacteriologist working for the CIA and was charged with developing bioweapons and delivery systems at Fort Detrick, Maryland. In 1953, Olson was covertly dosed with LSD by his colleagues during a retreat at Deep Creek Lake in Maryland.[17] After this administration, Olson was agitated and paranoid according to family and coworkers. Nine days after being dosed, Olson died after falling from a window of the Hotel Statler in New York City.[18] His death was initially ruled as a suicide, but subsequent investigations and reports, including those by his family, have suggested foul play or severe psychological distress induced by the LSD as contributing factors. Olson's case has become emblematic of the ethical breaches and human costs associated with MK-Ultra's experiments.

---

[15] Kinzer, S. (2019). *Poisoner in Chief.* Henry Holt. pp. 31, 53–54.

[16] Weinstein, H. (October 1, 1990). *Psychiatry and the CIA: Victims of Mind Control.* Amer Psychiatric Pub Inc.

[17] Regis, Ed. (1999). *The Biology of Doom: America's Secret Germ Warfare Project.* New York: Henry Holt & Company.

[18] Kinzer, S. (2019). From mind control to murder? How a deadly fall revealed the CIA's darkest secrets". *The Guardian* – via www.theguardian.com.

Drug Experiments

The CIA's interest in drugs for mind control led to extensive experimentation with LSD as the most prominent example. Beyond LSD, the experiments included a wide array of psychoactive and hallucinogenic substances:

- **LSD**: Intended to explore its potential for mind control and interrogation, subjects were often dosed without their knowledge. One infamous operation is known as "Operation Midnight Climax." This operation ran from 1954 to 1966 and it involved administering LSD to unsuspecting individuals in CIA safehouses. The goal of this experiment was to discover a way to protect US agents from clandestine interrogation methods and to surreptitiously gain control over enemy spies. In this project, prostitutes were employed to solicit unsuspecting men to have sex with them in CIA safehouses in New York City and San Francisco. After having sex with the subjects, the prostitutes were instructed to question them to see if the victims could be convinced to reveal personal secrets involuntarily. The "subjects" were given several different substances in the food or drink they were served before having sex, including psilocybin, mescaline, THC, and LSD. The effects of these drugs on the subject's ability and willingness to share information about themselves were monitored by the agents and the types of drugs and dosages were adjusted accordingly. CIA agents observed these interactions through a two-way mirror while recording them on film.[19] The outcomes of Midnight Climax experiments were never officially published, but anecdotal evidence from those overseeing the experiments provides some understanding of their effects. George Hunter White, an agent with the Federal Bureau of Narcotics, and Ira "Ike" Feldman, a former military intelligence officer who supervised experiments in San Francisco, observed that subjects became significantly more talkative under the combined

---

[19] (UNTITLED) | CIA FOIA (foia.cia.gov). *www.cia.gov*. Retrieved 2/7/24.

influence of drugs and sexual encounters.[20] There was no medical follow-up with these test subjects. The current whereabouts and condition of these human test subjects remain unknown, as does the full extent of any long-term effects they might have experienced.[21]

- **Mescaline and Psilocybin**: Derived from peyote cacti and psychedelic mushrooms, respectively, these substances were tested for their ability to induce altered states of consciousness and susceptibility to suggestion.

- **Barbiturates and Amphetamines**: In a technique known as the "barbiturate-amphetamine cocktail," subjects were injected with a barbiturate into one arm and an amphetamine into the other. The "barbiturate-amphetamine cocktail" technique, utilized within the scope of the CIA's MK-Ultra program, was an experimental interrogation method that sought to exploit the contrasting effects of two different classes of drugs to break down a subject's resistance and extract information. This method is also sometimes referred to as the "truth serum" approach, although its effectiveness at improving interrogations and ethical implications have been subjects of controversy.[22,23]

The barbiturates used in these experiments act as central nervous system depressants, inducing a state of sedation or inhibition. By injecting a barbiturate into one arm, the interrogators aimed to put the subject into a more relaxed, suggestible state, lowering their defenses and inhibitions against revealing information.

In contrast, amphetamines are stimulants that increase alertness and energy. Administering an amphetamine into the other arm was intended to counteract the sedative effects of the barbiturate, bringing the subject to a state of heightened alertness and, theoretically,

[20] Kinzer, S. (2019). *Poisoner in Chief; Sidney Gottlieb and the CIA Search for Mind Control.* New York: Henry Holt and Co, p. 149–51.

[21] MIND-BENDING DISCLOSURES | CIA FOIA (foia.cia.gov). *www.cia.gov.* Retrieved 2/7/24.

[22] Legge, D. and Steinberg, H. (1962). Actions of a mixture of amphetamine and a barbiturate in man. *Br J Pharmacol Chemother.* 18(3):490–500. doi: 10.1111/j.1476-5381.1962. tb01170.x.

[23] "Truth" drugs in Interrogation. chrome-extension://efaidnbmnnnibpcajpcglclefindmkaj/ https://www.cia.gov/resources/csi/static/Truth-Drugs-in-Interrogation.pdf (Accessed 6/14/24).

making them more susceptible to questioning and more likely to divulge information.

Either drug used alone, especially in a non-medical setting, is dangerous and can affect breathing, heart rate, and blood pressure. Either drug, if used inexpertly, can be fatal. The use of both drugs together had unknown consequences, especially in an uncontrolled and adversarial circumstance like an interrogation. And yet, they were administered frequently.

Specific instances of the use of the "barbiturate-amphetamine cocktail" are less well-documented in the public domain due to the classified nature of MK-Ultra and the subsequent destruction of many records related to the program in the 1970s. However, the existence of such programs has been acknowledged in declassified documents and reports that emerged following investigations into MK-Ultra, such as those conducted by the Church Committee in the mid-1970s.[24]

- **Hypnosis**: Hypnosis was a significant area of interest for the CIA as part of its broader effort to develop effective mind control.[25] The agency's fascination with hypnosis was driven by the potential to manipulate memory, elicit information, and potentially control actions without the subject's conscious awareness. This exploration was multifaceted, involving several key areas.

One of the primary goals was to determine if hypnosis could compel individuals to perform specific actions against their will or without their conscious knowledge.[26,27] This included acts of espionage, sabotage, and even the possibility of turning a subject into an unwitting assassin. The CIA was interested in whether a person could be hypnotically programmed to carry out complex instructions, such as

---

[24] https://www.senate.gov/about/powers-procedures/investigations/church-committee.htm (Accessed 2/9/24).

[25] https://web.archive.org/web/20190404095213/https://www.cia.gov/library/center-for-the-study-of-intelligence/kent-csi/vol4no1/html/v04i1a05p_0001.htm, retrieved 2/7/24.

[26] Reiter, P.J. (1958). *Antisocial or Criminal Acts and Hypnosis: A Case Study*. Springfield, Ill.: Charles C. Thomas.

[27] Schneck, J.M. (1947) A military offense induced by hypnosis. *J. Nervment. Dis.* 106, 186–189.

planting a bomb or stealing sensitive documents, and then have no recollection of the act or the programming itself.[28]

Hypnosis was also explored as a tool to enhance interrogation.[29] The idea was to use hypnotic induction to lower the subject's psychological defenses, making them more susceptible to suggestion and more likely to divulge secrets or confidential information. Interrogators experimented with hypnosis to bypass the conscious mind's resistance mechanisms, aiming for a direct line to the subconscious where hidden memories and information might be stored.

A critical aspect of the hypnotic experiments was the manipulation of memory. This included efforts to both implant false memories and erase or suppress real ones. The CIA was particularly interested in the potential to create amnesic barriers, using hypnosis to make subjects forget specific events, information, or even the fact that they had been hypnotized. This capability was seen as valuable for both operational security (e.g., ensuring subjects could not reveal sensitive information even if captured) and for erasing evidence of the mind control experiments themselves.

Understanding the variability in subjects' susceptibility to hypnosis was another area of investigation.[30] Not all individuals are equally susceptible to hypnotic induction, and the CIA conducted experiments to identify traits or conditions that made some people more receptive to hypnosis. This research aimed to refine selection criteria for subjects and to develop methods that could be used to increase susceptibility in less responsive individuals.

While the specific outcomes of hypnosis experiments under MK-Ultra are less documented in the public domain compared to other aspects of the program, the overarching nature of MK-Ultra's experiments suggests that subjects could have experienced harm. The full extent of harm caused by the MK-Ultra hypnosis experiments,

---

[28] https://www.cia.gov/readingroom/document/06760269 (Accessed 2/9/24).

[29] https://web.archive.org/web/20190404095213/https://www.cia.gov/library/center-for-the-study-of-intelligence/kent-csi/vol4no1/html/v04i1a05p_0001.htm#9-estabrooks-g-h (Accessed 2/7/24).

[30] Estabrooks, G.H. (1943). *Hypnotism*. New York: E. P. Dutton & Co., Inc.

like much of the program, remains partially obscured due to the classified nature of the project and the destruction of documents ordered by the CIA in the early 1970s. However, the revelations that have emerged from declassified documents, congressional investigations like the Church Committee, and accounts from participants and researchers have highlighted the program's disregard for ethical standards and the potential for harm to subjects. The psychological impact of being subjected to intense and manipulative hypnosis sessions, particularly without informed consent or understanding of the procedures, could include anxiety, stress, confusion, and a sense of loss of control. When hypnosis was used in conjunction with other MK-Ultra techniques like drug administration or sensory manipulation, the potential for harm increased, with subjects possibly experiencing long-lasting psychological trauma or alterations in their mental health.

Today, the idea that hypnosis can force someone to act against their deep-seated beliefs or will is considered more myth than reality. Its current use in therapy is to emphasize support and positive change rather than coercion.

- **Sensory Deprivation**: During a discussion of Soviet "brainwashing", Canadian Neuropsychologist Donald Hebb suggested in 1951 that the complete removal of sensory or perceptual stimulation might place someone 'in such a position psychologically that they would be susceptible to implantation of new or different ideas.'[31] The CIA sensory deprivation experiments aimed to explore the effects of removing stimuli on the human mind, with the goal of developing enhanced interrogation methods that could break down resistance.

The exploration of sensory deprivation by the CIA under programs like MK-Ultra delved into the psychological impacts of reducing or eliminating sensory inputs. These experiments were part of a broader attempt to understand and manipulate the human mind for

---

[31] Mccoy A. (2007) Science in Dachau's shadow: Hebb, beecher, and the development of CIA psychological torture and modern medical ethics. *Journal of the History of the Behavioral Sciences*. 43(4): 401–417. Published online in Wiley Interscience (www. interscience.wiley.com). doi: 10.1002/jhbs.20271 © 2007 Wiley Periodicals, Inc.

intelligence purposes. While the stated goal was to develop more effective interrogation abilities, the methods employed often crossed ethical boundaries, subjecting participants to extreme conditions that could be considered abusive or cruel. During these experiments, some subjects were placed in isolation for extended periods, which could last days or even weeks.

The use of isolation tanks was one of the more extreme forms of sensory deprivation explored. Subjects were placed in tanks designed to cut off all external stimuli: sight, sound, and touch were minimized by using body-temperature water to reduce the sensation of having a physical body and by soundproofing and darkening the tank. These sessions could last for hours or even days, leading to a range of psychological effects, including hallucinations, disorientation, and a heightened state of suggestibility. The prolonged lack of sensory input was sometimes used to break down individuals' psychological defenses, making them more amenable to interrogation or "reprogramming."

White Noise

Exposure to continuous white noise served as another method of sensory deprivation. Subjects were blindfolded to block out visual stimuli and then subjected to a constant, non-descript sound that masked auditory inputs. This technique aimed to disorient subjects and make them more susceptible to suggestion by creating a form of auditory isolation. The monotony and persistence of white noise could induce stress, anxiety, and disorientation, effects that interrogators hoped to leverage to break down resistance.

Beyond these methods, extended solitary confinement in specially designed cells that minimized sensory input was also explored. These environments were often devoid of natural light, with controlled temperature settings to reduce the sense of touch and spatial awareness.

These experiments often had profound and lasting psychological impacts on subjects. The prolonged lack of social interaction, visual and auditory stimulation, and the monotony of a featureless environment could lead to a range of psychological distress, including anxiety, hallucinations, and a breakdown of the sense of self.[32] In some cases, prolonged sensory deprivation can lead to psychotic-like experiences.[33] Reports of long-term effects include mental health issues, such as post-traumatic stress disorder (PTSD), anxiety, and depression.[34]

Environmental Manipulation

The manipulation of environmental factors to study their effects on human behavior was a significant aspect of the experiments conducted under programs like MK-Ultra. By altering room sizes and shapes, controlling light and sound levels, and rearranging objects and furniture, researchers aimed to disorient subjects and observe their reactions to confusion and stress. This approach was based on the hypothesis that environmental conditions could significantly impact psychological states and could be leveraged to develop interrogation methods for breaking down resistance.

Researchers experimented with changing the physical dimensions and configurations of rooms to study their psychological impact. For example, subjects might be placed in unusually shaped rooms with angled or curved walls that distorted their sense of space and orientation. The goal was to observe how disorientation affected their mental state and behavior.

Manipulating sensory inputs through light and sound was another common technique. Subjects could be exposed to varying levels of brightness or darkness, or to complete sensory deprivation, to study effects on mood and cognitive function. Similarly, sound levels could be adjusted from complete silence to overwhelming noise, including white noise or repetitive sounds, to induce stress or disorientation.

---

[32] Sahoo, S., Naskar, C., Singh, A., Rijal, R., Mehra, A. and Grover, S. (2022). Sensory Deprivation and Psychiatric Disorders: Association, Assessment and Management Strategies. *Indian J Psychol Med.* 44(5):436–444. doi: 10.1177/02537176211033920. Epub 2021 Sep 21.

[33] Daniel, C. and Mason, O.J. (2015). Predicting psychotic-like experiences during sensory deprivation. *Biomed Res Int.* 2015:439379. doi: 10.1155/2015/439379. Epub 2015 Feb 24.

[34] Raz, M. (2013), Alone again: John Zubek and the troubled history of sensory deprivation research. *J. Hist. Behav. Sci.* 49: 379–395. https://doi.org/10.1002/jhbs.21631.

The arrangement of objects and furniture was altered to create unfamiliar or confusing environments. Subjects might find themselves in rooms where furniture was placed in unexpected positions, or where objects were arranged in a way that defied normal logic or function, challenging their ability to adapt and respond to new and disorienting situations.

The public became aware of the MK-Ultra program primarily through investigative journalism and the efforts of the U.S. government to investigate and expose illegal and unethical activities conducted by its intelligence agencies. The pivotal moment came in the 1970s, following a series of events that brought to light the extent of the CIA's involvement in mind control experiments and other covert operations.

Ethical Breaches of MK-Ultra and Project ARTICHOKE

The MK-Ultra and Project ARTICHOKE programs, initiated during the Cold War era, are now infamously known for their significant ethical violations, which have had a lasting impact on the field of medical and psychological research ethics. These programs, driven by the United States government's ambition to master mind control and counter perceived global threats, conducted experiments that ranged from the administration of psychoactive drugs, including LSD, to hypnosis, sensory deprivation, and a variety of other procedures, often on unwitting subjects. The ethical breaches committed in the name of national security raise profound questions about the limits of scientific inquiry and the responsibilities of researchers:

Lack of Informed Consent: A fundamental ethical violation was the lack of informed consent. Many subjects of these experiments were not aware they were part of a study, much less informed of the potential risks or the nature of the research they were subjected to. This disregard for autonomy undermines the ethical foundation of voluntary participation in research.

Deliberate Deception: Closely related to the lack of informed consent was the deliberate deception of research subjects. Participants were often misled about the nature of the experiments, or completely unaware they were part of a study, violating the trust placed in researchers and institutions by participants and society. This deception not only compromised the integrity of the research relationship but also exposed subjects to unknown risks without their knowledge or consent.

Exposure to Harm: The experiments frequently exposed subjects to significant psychological and physical risks without their consent or sometimes even their knowledge. The administration of drugs like LSD, practices of sensory deprivation, and other forms of psychological stress could have long-lasting effects on an individual's mental health and well-being. The cruelty of these experiments lies not only in the physical and psychological discomfort experienced by the subjects but also in the lasting damage to their mental health and well-being. The ethical principle of minimizing harm — ensuring that research does not harm participants and that any potential risks are clearly outweighed by the benefits — was violated in these cases.

The revelations about these ethical breaches contributed to a reevaluation of ethical standards in research, leading to the establishment of more rigorous guidelines and oversight mechanisms, such as IRBs in the United States. Discussing the ethical violations of MK-Ultra and Project ARTICHOKE is crucial not only for understanding a dark chapter in American history but also for appreciating the evolution of ethical standards in medical and psychological research. Today, the legacy of these programs serves as a cautionary tale about the potential for abuse when scientific research is conducted without stringent ethical oversight and transparency, highlighting the importance of ethical vigilance and the need to balance scientific curiosity with the imperative to protect the rights and dignity of individuals.

Inquiry and Public Revelation

While not directly related to MK-Ultra, the Watergate scandal of the early 1970s played a significant role in fostering a climate of skepticism and critical examination of government activities. The scandal's exposure of illegal activities within the Nixon administration led to increased scrutiny of other government agencies, including the CIA.

In 1974, investigative journalist Seymour Hersh published a series of articles in *The New York Times* revealing the CIA's illegal domestic activities, including spying on American citizens and conducting unauthorized experiments.[35] Although Hersh's articles did not specifically name MK-Ultra, they contributed to a growing demand for transparency and accountability within the intelligence community.

The passage and subsequent amendments of the Freedom of Information Act (FOIA) provided journalists, researchers, and the general public with a mechanism to request and obtain government documents. FOIA requests led to the release of thousands of documents related to MK-Ultra, offering concrete evidence of the program's existence and the scope of its experiments.

In response to the revelations and public outcry, the U.S. Senate established the Church Committee in 1975, formally known as the United States Senate Select Committee to Study Governmental Operations with Respect to Intelligence Activities. Chaired by Senator Frank Church,[36] the committee conducted a thorough investigation into the activities of the CIA, FBI, NSA, and other intelligence agencies. The investigation was hindered by both a lack of records and cooperative witnesses. As Senator Edward Kennedy said during his opening remarks at the Church Committee hearings,

"Perhaps most disturbing of all was the fact that the extent of experimentation on human subjects was unknown. The records of all these activities were destroyed in January 1973 at the instruction of then-CIA Director Richard Helms. Despite persistent inquiries by both the Health Subcommittee and the Intelligence

---

[35] https://www.nytimes.com/1974/12/22/archives/huge-cia-operation-reported-in-u-s-against-antiwar-forces-other.html (Accessed 2/9/24).

[36] Frank Forrester Church III was an American politician and a lawyer. A member of the Democratic Party, he served as a United States senator from Idaho from 1957 until his defeat in 1980. He was the chairman of the Senate Foreign Relations Committee.

Committee, no additional records or information were forthcoming. And no one — no single individual — could be found who remembered the details, not the Director of the CIA, who ordered the documents destroyed, not the official responsible for the program, nor any of his associates."[37]

Despite this, during its investigation, the committee uncovered details about MK-Ultra and other programs aimed at mind control and enhanced interrogation. They confirmed that the CIA had conducted extensive experiments on humans to develop interrogation and mind control under MK-Ultra, Project ARTICHOKE, and related programs. The committee's reports highlighted significant ethical and legal violations, including breaches of informed consent, deception, and exposure of participants to harm.

The combination of investigative journalism, legislative inquiry, and legal mechanisms for obtaining government documents culminated in the exposure of MK-Ultra to the public. This exposure not only revealed the extent of the CIA's involvement in unethical research practices but also prompted significant reforms in the oversight of intelligence activities and the protection of human subjects in research.

Impact and Legacy of MK-Ultra and Project ARTICHOKE

The MK-Ultra and Project ARTICHOKE programs, despite being shrouded in secrecy for many years, have left a profound and indelible mark on the fields of medical and psychological research, as well as on public awareness and policy regarding ethical standards in human experimentation. The revelation of these programs and their controversial experiments significantly influenced the evolution of ethical guidelines and the establishment of oversight mechanisms designed to protect the rights and dignity of research subjects.

---

[37] http://www.druglibrary.org/schaffer/history/e1950/mkultra/Hearing01.htm.

- **Reevaluation of Ethical Standards**: The exposure of the ethical breaches committed by MK-Ultra and Project ARTICHOKE — ranging from the lack of informed consent and deliberate deception to the exposure of participants to harm — prompted a critical reevaluation of the ethical standards governing research involving human subjects. The public outcry and subsequent scrutiny highlighted the necessity of stringent ethical oversight in scientific research, particularly research funded or conducted by government agencies.

- **Establishment of IRBs**: One of the most significant outcomes of the revelations about MK-Ultra and Project ARTICHOKE was the establishment of IRBs in the United States. Mandated by the National Research Act of 1974, IRBs are tasked with reviewing research proposals involving human subjects to ensure compliance with ethical standards. This includes evaluating the risks and benefits of the research, ensuring informed consent is obtained, and monitoring the research to protect participants from harm.

- **Influence on Ethical Guidelines**: The legacy of these programs also contributed to the development and reinforcement of ethical guidelines for research, such as the Belmont Report, published in 1979. The Belmont Report established key ethical principles for research involving human subjects, including respect for persons (autonomy), beneficence (do no harm and maximize benefits), and justice (fairness in distribution). These principles have become foundational in research ethics, guiding researchers and IRBs in the ethical conduct of studies.

- **Public Awareness and Policy Changes**: The MK-Ultra and Project ARTICHOKE programs have also had a lasting impact on public awareness and policy regarding government-sponsored research. The scandal underscored the potential for abuse when research lacks transparency and accountability, leading to increased demands for public oversight of intelligence and research activities. Policy changes, including reforms within the CIA and other intelligence agencies, were implemented to prevent future abuses.

Today, the legacy of MK-Ultra and Project ARTICHOKE serves as a cautionary tale about the potential for abuse in scientific research, especially when conducted under the auspices of national security. It underscores the importance of ethical vigilance, the protection of individual rights in research, and the need for a balance between scientific curiosity and ethical responsibility. The programs have become a pivotal story in the history of medical and psychological research ethics, reminding researchers, policymakers, and the public of the critical importance of maintaining ethical standards to protect the well-being of all research participants.

Despite the ethical and legal issues surrounding the MK-Ultra program and Gottlieb's central role in it, he and his colleagues were never prosecuted for their involvement in the experiments. The covert nature of the program, along with the destruction of many MK-Ultra documents in 1973 on Gottlieb's orders, complicated efforts to hold individuals accountable. The revelations about MK-Ultra and other CIA activities led to congressional investigations, but these did not result in criminal charges against Gottlieb or other key figures. Gottlieb remained the head of MK-Ultra and was awarded the Distinguish Intelligence Medal.[38] He retired from the CIA in 1973. Afterward, he traveled frequently, earned a master's degree in speech pathology, and spent time in his home in Virginia. He died peacefully at home on March 7, 1999, at the age of 80.

The Olson family threatened to sue the government over Frank Olson's "wrongful death" in 1975. This legal action was prompted by revelations about the circumstances surrounding Olson's death and his involvement in CIA experiments. Fearing further embarrassing revelations, the government made a settlement offer of $750,000 ($4,276,198.88 in 2024 dollars) and subsequent personal apologies from President Gerald Ford and CIA Director William Colby. Both were accepted.

The Effect of MK-Ultra on Therapeutic LSD Research

LSD was created by the Swiss chemist Albert Hofmann in 1938.[39] Hofmann initially synthesized LSD while searching for ergot derivatives

---

[38] https://www.theguardian.com/news/1999/mar/11/guardianobituaries2.

[39] Stoll, A., Hofmann, A. Partialsynthese von Alkaloiden vom Typus des Ergobasins. (6. Mitteilung über Mutterkornalkaloide). (1943). *Helv Chim Acta.* 26:944–5. doi: 10.1002/hlca.19430260326.

that could help reduce postpartum hemorrhage. A few years later, Hofmann accidentally exposed himself to a small dose of LSD, becoming the first person to experience its potent effects.[40] By the late 1940s, psychiatrists had begun to show significant interest in LSD's potential as a therapeutic tool.[41] It was during the 1950s that Sandoz Laboratories began marketing LSD under the brand name "Delysid,"[42] and it was subsequently used in numerous psychiatric departments across Europe and America. LSD was touted in the media as a revolutionary psychiatric medicine.[43] One author, after analyzing 25,000 therapy sessions using LSD, concluded that "with the proper precautions, psychedelics are safe." Indeed, from 1950 to the mid-1960s, the field of psychedelic drug therapy witnessed significant scholarly activity, with over a thousand clinical papers covering 40,000 patients, numerous books, and 6 international conferences dedicated to the subject. This burgeoning interest in psychedelic therapy attracted many psychiatrists who were not necessarily cultural rebels or particularly radical in their professional outlook.[44]

However, the use of LSD in programs like MK-Ultra was a significant factor in the growing concerns and subsequent restriction of LSD. The revelation of MK-Ultra and similar projects to the public, particularly the unethical administration of LSD without consent, contributed to a significant outcry and concern over the safety and control of psychoactive substances. The association of LSD with government-sponsored mind control experiments added to the drug's controversial image and raised ethical and safety concerns among the public and lawmakers.

---

[40] Hofmann, A., and Feilding, A., (2013). eds. LSD: My problem child and insights/outlooks. In: *J. Ott, Trans.* Oxford University Press: New York, NY, US.

[41] Busch, A.K. and Johnson, W.C. (1950). L.S.D. 25 as an aid in psychotherapy; preliminary report of a new drug. *Dis Nerv Syst* 11:241–243.

[42] https://www.emcdda.europa.eu/publications/drug-profiles/lsd_en#:~:text=During%20the%201950s%20and%201960s,with%20the%20psychedelic%20period.

[43] Siff, S. (2015). *Acid Hype: American News Media and the Psychedelic Experience.* Urbana, Il: University of Illinois Press, p. 60.

[44] Grinspoon, L. and Bakalar, J.B. (1979) *Psychedelic Drugs Reconsidered*, Basic Books, New York, p. 192.

Media reports on MK-Ultra and other incidents involving LSD contributed to a moral panic[45] about the drug's use and effects. Sensationalized stories about LSD's dangers, including its role in MK-Ultra, fueled public fear and called for stricter regulations.

The idea that LSD could be used as a tool for mind control or psychological manipulation by foreign powers or within the United States contributed to the urgency of controlling the substance.

The widespread recreational use of LSD in the counterculture movement of the 1960s, which often challenged societal norms and authority, further alarmed the government and conservative elements of society. The government's efforts to restrict LSD were partly aimed at curbing what was seen as subversive behavior.

The culmination of these factors, including the ethical controversies surrounding MK-Ultra, played a role in the decision to classify LSD as a Schedule I drug under the Controlled Substances Act of 1970. The classification of LSD as a Schedule I drug, the most restrictive category of drugs, effectively ended legal clinical research on the substance for decades, despite its initial promise in psychiatric research and therapy. The decision was driven more by the sociopolitical climate of the time than by scientific consensus about the drug's medical utility or safety profile.

After LSD was classified as a Schedule I drug, research into its potential therapeutic uses, particularly for mental health disorders, faced significant regulatory and funding obstacles, leading to a substantial decline in scientific interest for the next 30 years.

Fortunately, starting in the late 1990s and early 2000s, there was a gradual resurgence of interest in the therapeutic potential of psychedelics, including LSD, for treating various conditions including treatment-resistant depression, anxiety disorders, post-traumatic stress disorder, substance

---

[45] Cohen, S. (1960). Lysergic Acid Diethylamide: Side Effects and Complications. *The Journal of Nervous and Mental Disease.* 130(1):30–40. https://doi.org/10.1097/00005053-196001000-00005.

abuse disorders, and cluster headaches.[46,47] Early-stage clinical trials utilizing LSD in these conditions have reported positive findings regarding its safety and efficacy.[48]

Conclusion

The MK-Ultra Program, with its clandestine sprawl into the depths of human consciousness, stands as a stark reminder of a period when the pursuit of knowledge and power eclipsed the fundamental principles of human rights and dignity. The revelations surrounding this program have not only shed light on a shadowy chapter of Cold War history but also forced a reckoning with the ethical boundaries of state-sponsored research. The legacy of MK-Ultra, far from being a mere historical footnote, has catalyzed a profound transformation in the oversight and conduct of research involving human subjects. It underscores the imperative for transparency, accountability, and, above all, respect for the individual, ensuring that the quest for advancement never again comes at the cost of our most basic ethical commitments.

---

[46] Müller, F., Mühlhauser, M., Holze, F., Lang, U.E., Walter, M., Liechti, M.E. and Borgwardt, S. (2020). Treatment of a Complex Personality Disorder Using Repeated Doses of LSD—A Case Report on Significant Improvements in the Absence of Acute Drug Effects, Frontiers in Psychiatry, 11, URL: =https://www.frontiersin.org/journals/psychiatry/articles/10.3389/fpsyt.2020.573953.

[47] Fuentes, J.J., Fonseca, F., Elices, M. and Farré, M., and Torrens M. (Jan 21 2020). Therapeutic use of LSD in psychiatry: A systematic review of randomized-controlled clinical trials. *Front Psychiatry*. 10: 943. doi: 10.3389/fpsyt.2019.00943. PMID: 32038315; PMCID: PMC6985449.

[48] Nichols, D.E. (2016). Psychedelics. *Pharmacol Rev.*, 68(2): 264–355. doi: 10.1124/pr.115.011478. Erratum in: *Pharmacol Rev.*, 68(2):356. PMID: 26841800; PMCID: PMC4813425.

Further Reading

For those interested in exploring the depths of the MK-Ultra program and its implications on mind control and psychological experimentation, here is a curated list of books that delve into this secretive chapter of history:

1. **"MK-ULTRA: The CIA's Top Secret Program in Human Experimentation and Behavior Modification" by George Andrews, PhD**
   - This book provides an in-depth look into the CIA's top-secret program focused on human experimentation and behavior modification.

2. **"Brainwash: The Secret History of Mind Control" by Dominic Streatfeild, Thomas Dunne Books, First Edition (March 6, 2007)**
   - While not exclusively about MK-Ultra, this book offers a broader perspective on mind control's secret history, including insights into the MK-Ultra program.

3. **"Project MK-Ultra and Mind Control Technology: A Compilation of Patents and Reports" by Alex Baalthazar, Adventures Unlimited Press (June 14, 2017)**
   - This compilation provides a technical perspective on the mind control technology developed under Project MK-Ultra, featuring patents and reports related to the program.

4. **"The Search for the Manchurian Candidate: The CIA and Mind Control" by Marks, John D. (1979), New York Times Books**
   - This book provides a comprehensive history of MK-Ultra and related programs, based on documents obtained through the FOIA and interviews with participants.

5. **"Mind Wars: Brain Science and the Military in the 21st Century" by Moreno, Jonathan D. (2013), Bellevue Literary Press**
   - Moreno discusses the legacy of MK-Ultra in the context of modern military and intelligence research into brain science, offering insights into ethical considerations.

6. **"Journey into Madness: The True Story of Secret CIA Mind Control and Medical Abuse" by Thomas, Gordon (1989), Bantam**
   - This work offers a detailed account of the experiments and their impact on subjects, with a focus on the ethical breaches involved.

Church Committee Reports (1976) Official title: "Final Report of the Select Committee to Study Governmental Operations with Respect to Intelligence Activities, United States Senate"

- These reports contain extensive documentation on MK-Ultra, Project ARTICHOKE, and other CIA activities. They are available in full through the U.S. Government Printing Office or online archives like the Digital National Security Archive.

Freedom of Information Act (FOIA) Documents

- The CIA has declassified a significant number of documents related to MK-Ultra and Project ARTICHOKE, which can be found through the CIA's FOIA Electronic Reading Room or the Black Vault, an online repository of declassified government documents.

Ethical Guidelines

The Nuremberg Code (1947)

- As one of the earliest sets of guidelines for ethical research conduct, the principles outlined in the Nuremberg Code are directly relevant to the ethical analysis of MK-Ultra and Project ARTICHOKE.

World Medical Association (1964): Declaration of Helsinki

- This declaration is a key document in medical ethics, providing guidelines for research involving human subjects. It's useful for discussing the ethical standards that were violated by the experiments.

Online Archives and Databases

- Digital National Security Archive
- CIA's FOIA Electronic Reading Room
- The Black Vault

Chapter 8

Montreal Experiments

In the annals of psychological research, the Montreal Experiments conducted by Dr. Donald Ewen Cameron represent a dark and controversial chapter marked by egregious ethical violations and profound human suffering. Operating under the guise of advancing psychiatric treatment, Cameron's experiments at the Allan Memorial Institute, funded in part by the CIA, subjected unwitting patients to extreme and unproven methods of mind control and behavior modification. These individuals, seeking help for common psychiatric ailments, became instead subjects of experiments in mind control. They were exposed to a horrifying array of treatments including electroshock therapy at intensities far beyond the therapeutic standard, drug-induced comas, psychic driving, and sensory deprivation. The aftermath of these experiments left many patients with irreversible damage, including severe memory loss, psychological distress, and an inability to function independently. Cameron's work, driven by a blend of scientific curiosity and Cold War-era motivations, not only breached the fundamental principles of medical ethics and human rights but also inflicted untold horror on those placed under his care. This chapter delves into the chilling details of Cameron's experiments, highlighting the stark ethical breaches and the lasting impact on the victims and the field of psychiatric research.

Dr. Donald Ewen Cameron (Figure 1) was a Scottish-born psychiatrist who played a controversial role in the history of psychological research due to his experiments in Montreal, Canada, during the 1950s and early 1960s. Cameron was one of the most prominent psychiatrists in North

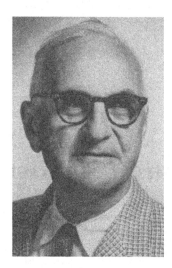

Figure 1.   Dr. Donald Ewen Cameron.

Source: Image public domain.

America as well as a former president of both the Canadian and American psychiatric associations[1,2] and he served as the director of the psychiatric hospital at the Allan Memorial Institute. The Allen Memorial Hospital is part of the Royal Victoria Hospital and is affiliated with McGill University. His tenure at the Allan Memorial Institute spanned from 1943 to 1964, during which time he conducted his controversial experiments.

With funding from the CIA, he performed a series of mind-control experiments on hundreds of people between 1957 and 1961.[3] The patients in this experiment had entered the Allan Institute voluntarily, usually at the recommendation of a private physician. These experiments involved a wide range of patients, many of whom were seeking treatment for

---

[1] Zilboorg, G. (1953). "D. Ewen Cameron M.D., President, 1952-1953: A Biographical Sketch". *American Journal of Psychiatry*. 110(1): 10–12. doi: 10.1176/ajp.110.1.10.

[2] Past Presidents & Board Chairs – Canadian Psychiatric Association – Association des psychiatres du Canada. *Canadian Psychiatric Association – Association des psychiatres du Canada*. Retrieved 2018-05-10. https://www.cpa-apc.org/about-cpa/who-we-are/past-presidents-board-chairs/ (Accessed 6/14/24).

[3] https://www.washingtonpost.com/archive/lifestyle/1985/07/28/25-years-of-nightmares/cb836420-9c72-4d3c-ae60-70a8f13c4ceb/ (Accessed 6/14/24).

common psychiatric disorders, such as depression, anxiety, and postpartum depression. Some patients were admitted for issues that would be considered relatively minor by today's standards, such as anxiety, marital difficulties, or chronic fatigue. The diversity in the patient population was significant, with individuals varying in age, background, and the severity of their conditions.

Cameron's motivations for these experiments were rooted in his theories about mental illness and the potential for "reprogramming" the human mind. He believed that certain psychiatric conditions could be treated by erasing harmful patterns of behavior and thought and then rebuilding the psyche in a healthier manner.[4] This approach was based on his broader interest in the structure of the psyche and the possibility of influencing it through external stimuli.

Cameron was driven by a desire to find new treatments for mental illnesses that were resistant to existing therapies. He theorized that by breaking down existing patterns of behavior and thought (depatterning), he could create a "clean slate" upon which healthier patterns could be established.[5]

Cameron was also motivated by a broader scientific curiosity about the workings of the human mind and the potential for controlling or altering its functions. His work was innovative and radical for its time, pushing the boundaries of what was known about psychological conditioning and therapy.

The broader context of the Cold War and the race for psychological and technological superiority likely influenced Cameron's work. His experiments received funding from the CIA as part of MK-Ultra, indicating an interest from the U.S. government in exploring the potential of psychological techniques for interrogation and mind control. This funding may have provided both financial resources and a sense of urgency or importance to his research. Dr. Cameron's experiments focused on mind control, behavior modification, and the exploration of potential

---

[4] https://aeon.co/ideas/the-history-of-brainwashing-is-a-red-flag-for-techno-therapy (Accessed 2/13/24).
[5] https://www.sciencedirect.com/science/article/abs/pii/S0010440X62800157 (Accessed 6/14/24).

treatments for mental illness. Here's a description of the key components of his experiments:

Breaking Down and Rebuilding the Psyche

One of Cameron's most notorious techniques was "psychic driving." In 1953, he developed the theory of psychic driving in which a patient's mind could be manipulated using verbal cues played repeatedly.[6,7] He believed he could erase harmful patterns of behavior and thought, allowing for new, healthier patterns to be created.

This process involved two phases: depatterning and psychic driving.

Depatterning: Dr. Cameron used electroshock therapy to erase and alter the memories of patients. Electroconvulsive therapy (ECT), also known as electroshock therapy, is a medical procedure employed to treat psychological conditions, such as treatment-resistant depression.[8] In modern psychiatric care, the treatment parameters, including duration, voltage, and amperage, are carefully controlled and individualized based on the patient's needs and response to treatment. Modern ECT machines are designed to deliver a precise, brief electrical stimulus, and the focus is more on the control of electrical charge and current rather than the voltage alone. The goal is to induce a therapeutic seizure with the minimum necessary electrical charge to achieve the desired clinical effect while minimizing side effects. A typical series of treatments could range from 4 to 20 sessions to treat severe depression. Most people need 6–12 treatments, usually given 2–3 times a week for 3–4 weeks. The number of treatments depends on the severity of symptoms and how quickly they respond to treatment.

However, in Dr. Cameron's experiments, an intensive form of ECT was utilized as a method for brain depatterning.[9] Typically, patients

---

[6] Cameron, D.E. (1956). Psychic driving. *American Journal of Psychiatry*, 112(7): 502–509.
[7] Ewen, D.C. (1960). Production of differential amnesia as a factor in the treatment of schizophrenia. *Comprehensive Psychiatry*, 1(1):26–34, ISSN 0010-440X, https://doi.org/10.1016/S0010-440X(60)80047-8. (https://www.sciencedirect.com/science/article/pii/S0010440X60800478).
[8] "Electroconvulsive therapy (ECT) - Mayo Clinic". *www.mayoclinic.org*. Retrieved 2.12.24.
[9] "The Secret Montreal Experiments They Don't Want You To Know About". Retrieved 2/7/24.

underwent 2–3 sessions daily, each session delivering 6 shocks of 150 volts for one second. These shocks were delivered at 75 times the usual intensity.[10] This regimen continued for 30–40 days. Subsequently, researchers gradually decreased the frequency of the sessions, concluding the treatment with a two-year follow-up program that included one session per month. This was intended to break down the patient's existing mental state, reducing them to a more childlike condition.

In addition to ECT, patients were often sedated with a cocktail of drugs to promote "depatterning." Cameron's protocol for using sedative drugs involved administering a combination of powerful sedatives and other psychoactive substances to patients over extended periods, often lasting several weeks. This regimen was designed to induce a prolonged state of sedation or sleep, during which the patient's brain was believed to be more receptive to reprogramming. The drugs commonly used in this protocol included the following:

- **Barbiturates**: These were used to sedate patients deeply, often to the point of inducing a coma-like state.
- **Insulin Coma Therapy**: High doses of insulin were administered to produce hypoglycemia and, subsequently, coma. Patients would be brought out of this state with glucose injections. While ultimately ineffective, Insulin Coma Therapy was associated with seizures, permanent neurological damage, and a 1% mortality rate.[11]
- **LSD and Other Psychoactive Drugs**: Cameron experimented with a variety of psychoactive drugs as part of his treatments, including LSD, PCP, insulin, and barbiturates. LSD was of particular interest, given its powerful hallucinogenic effects, which Cameron believed could be used to access and alter the subconscious mind. Patients under this treatment were kept in isolated rooms, sometimes restrained to their beds, to prevent self-harm and to ensure the controlled delivery of the audio messages that were part of the psychic driving process.

---

[10] https://www.washingtonpost.com/archive/lifestyle/1985/07/28/25-years-of-nightmares/cb836420-9c72-4d3c-ae60-70a8f13c4ceb/?_pml=1 (Accessed 6/14/24).

[11] chrome-extension://efaidnbmnnnibpcajpcglclefindmkaj/https://www.ncbi.nlm.nih.gov/pmc/articles/PMC1297956/pdf/10741319.pdf (Accessed 6/14/24).

- **Drug-Induced Sleep**: Cameron also employed "drug-induced sleep" as a way of depatterning and repatterning the brains of subjects. In this experiment, patients were placed into an artificial coma using high doses of Thorazine. These sleep sessions lasted from a few days to 86 days. The patients weren't made aware of how long they would be asleep. The theoretical basis for this drug treatment was rooted in his belief in the necessity of breaking down existing mental patterns before new, healthier ones could be established.

- **Sensory Deprivation**: In addition to the drug regimen, patients might be subjected to sensory deprivation techniques to limit external distractions and focus their attention solely on the audio messages. Patients might be isolated in a room, cut off from sensory stimuli such as light, sound, and touch, to explore the effects of sensory deprivation on the psyche. This technique was based on the theory that removing external stimuli could make the mind more malleable and open to reprogramming. While short-term sessions of sensory deprivation may be relaxing and conducive to deep thought or meditation, extended or forced sensory deprivation can result in extreme anxiety, hallucinations,[12] bizarre thoughts, and depression.[13] To enhance the sensory deprivation, patients were given little food or water, and instead injected with drugs to confuse and paralyze them including LSD and, curare.[14]

Psychic Driving: In the second phase, patients were exposed to looped audio recordings made by Cameron or his staff. Patients would listen to these messages through headphones, sometimes while in a drug-induced sleep. The procedure involved playing these recorded messages for up to 16 hours daily for days on end. Throughout the entire duration, these

---

[12] Sireteanu, R., Oertel, V., Mohr, H., Linden, D. and Singer, W. (2008). Graphical illustration and functional neuroimaging of visual hallucinations during prolonged blindfolding: A comparison to visual imagery. *Perception*. 37(12): 1805–1821. doi: 10.1068/p6034.

[13] Stuart Grassian Psychiatric effects of solitary confinement (PDF). This article is a redacted, non-institution- and non-inmate-specific version of a declaration submitted in September 1993 in Madrid v. Gomez, 889F.Supp.1146.

[14] The Secret Montreal Experiments They Don't Want You To Know About". Retrieved 2/12/24.

messages could be replayed as many as half a million times in total. Initially, for the first 10 days, the recordings featured personal, negative messages. This phase was then succeeded by another 10 days during which the messages were positive.[15] The theory was that these messages would penetrate the patient's consciousness and lead to new patterns of thought and behavior. Patients sometimes objected to listening to the recordings, so Cameron put speakers in football helmets and locked them onto their heads. Often, patients would experience anxiety and agitation during these intense sessions, sometimes banging their heads into walls.[16] To manage this anxiety, patients were administered high doses of sedative drugs, including Sodium Amytal and Largactil.[17,18]

Outcomes

The outcomes of the psychic driving phase were mixed and often detrimental to the patients. These outcomes included the following:

- **Limited Success in Behavioral Modification**: While Cameron believed that psychic driving could effectively reprogram patients' behaviors and cure mental illnesses, there was little evidence to support its efficacy. The approach did not result in the desired therapeutic outcomes and, in many cases, left patients in a worse condition than before the treatment.
- **Memory Loss**: Many patients experienced significant memory loss, not only of the period during which they were treated but also of their lives before the treatment. This included losing memories of personal identity, family, skills, and knowledge. Louis Weinstein, a successful Canadian Businessman, entered the Allman Institute with complaints

[15] 1950s–1960s: Dr. Ewen Cameron Destroyed Minds at Allan Memorial Hospital in Montreal - AHRP. *AHRP*. 2015-01-18. Retrieved 2/7/24.

[16] https://www.theguardian.com/world/2018/may/03/montreal-brainwashing-allan-memorial-institute retrieved 2/12/2024.

[17] Donald Ewen Cameron. *Spartacus Educational*. Retrieved 2/7/24.

[18] Full text of "George Cooper Report Ewen Cameron, 1986. *archive.org*. 1986. Retrieved 2/7/24.

of respiratory and gastric complaints associated with stress and anxiety. After his treatment, he was completely changed. He'd lost his memory and couldn't care for himself or even carry on a conversation.[19,20] He could no longer work and needed to be cared for the rest of his life.

- **Psychological Distress**: The invasive and repetitive nature of the psychic driving technique caused considerable psychological distress for many patients. Reports of anxiety, confusion, and disorientation were common, with some individuals suffering long-term psychological effects.

In a 1956 study conducted by Cameron,[21] a tape recorder was utilized to capture the voice of a 40-year-old female patient repeating a deeply emotional phrase from her childhood: 'If you don't keep quiet, I'm going to leave you behind.' This phrase, originally spoken to her by her mother, had a lasting impact on her. The patient was then subjected to listening to this personal and distressing statement a total of 45 times. Throughout this process, she exhibited significant signs of emotional distress: she pleaded with the researcher to cease the playback, her face turned red, she began to hyperventilate, and she started to shake — a physical reaction that persisted even after the recording had stopped.

Velma Orlikow, another patient of Dr. Cameron, suffered from postpartum depression. After three years of depatterning therapy, which included the use of LSD and electroshock therapy, she was no longer the same patient. A former lover of books, she could no longer focus on even reading short articles. Letter writing was impossible. She became anxious and explosive in social situations.

- **Prosopagnosia**: Prosopagnosia is the inability to recognize faces. In one incident, a young intern named Mary Morrow approached Cameron seeking a fellowship in psychiatry. However, after a physical examination, Cameron deemed Morrow "tired and nervous" and said

---

[19] https://www.washingtonpost.com/archive/lifestyle/1985/07/28/25-years-of-nightmares/cb836420-9c72-4d3c-ae60-70a8f13c4ceb/?_pml=1 (Accessed 2/12/24).

[20] Weinstein, H.L. (1988). *A Father, a Son and the CIA.*

[21] Cameron, D.E (1956). Psychic driving. *American Journal of Psychiatry*, 112(7):502–509.

he would not consider her for a position unless she underwent "sleep therapy". Rather than getting a job, she was admitted as a patient. For 11 days, Morrow was subjected to de-patterning experiments, which involved electroshock therapy and barbiturates.[22] These treatments led to brain anoxia, a condition where the brain does not receive enough oxygen, necessitating her hospitalization. As a result of these experiments, Morrow now suffers from prosopagnosia, a condition that impairs her ability to recognize faces.

Ethical Concerns

Dr. Cameron's experiments have become infamous for their ethical violations, which starkly contravened the principles of medical ethics and human rights. These violations include the following.

One of the most egregious ethical breaches was the lack of informed consent. Many patients subjected to Cameron's experiments were not adequately informed about the nature, risks, and potential adverse effects of the treatments. In some cases, patients were led to believe they were receiving standard therapeutic care for their psychiatric conditions, without understanding they were part of experimental procedures that included unproven and potentially harmful techniques like psychic driving, prolonged drug-induced sleep, and excessive ECT.

Cameron's experiments often involved deliberate deception. Patients were not told the true purpose of the treatments they received nor were they aware that these were part of a broader research initiative funded by the CIA as part of MK-Ultra. This deception violated the ethical principle of respect for autonomy, undermining patients' ability to make informed decisions about their care.

The experimental protocols employed by Cameron exposed patients to significant harm, both psychological and physical. The use of high-dose ECT, psychoactive drugs like LSD, and prolonged periods of sensory deprivation or overload led to severe and sometimes irreversible damage. Patients reported long-term effects, such as memory loss, cognitive

---

[22] chrome-extension://efaidnbmnnnibpcajpcglclefindmkaj/https://www.cia.gov/reading room/docs/CIA-RDP88-01070R000301530003-5.pdf (Accessed 6/14/24).

impairment, emotional distress, and in some cases, a complete inability to function independently after the treatment. The principle of non-maleficence, which obligates medical professionals to "do no harm," was clearly violated.

Cameron's actions represented a breach of the professional duty of care owed to patients. The primary obligation of a physician is to act in the best interest of their patients, a duty that was fundamentally compromised by Cameron's focus on experimental research over patient welfare. This breach of trust has had lasting implications for the credibility of psychiatric research and the importance of ethical oversight in medical experiments.

The experiments conducted by Cameron disregarded the inherent dignity of the patients involved. Treating individuals as mere subjects for research without regard for their well-being or consent dehumanized them and violated their basic human rights. This aspect of Cameron's work highlights the need for ethical principles in research, including respect for persons and the recognition of their right to self-determination and protection from harm.

Of interest, Cameron was one of the psychiatrists present at the Nuremberg trials to evaluate the mental capability of the accused.[23] He met the architects of the holocaust and was made aware of their crimes. Cameron was appalled by the experiments conducted during World War II and he expressed his horror and reflections in a paper titled 'Nuremberg and its significance,' where he detailed the atrocities of these experiments and discussed their implications for the German people.[24]

Legacy and Reforms

The ethical violations associated with Dr. Cameron's experiments contributed to significant reforms in research ethics, including the establishment of Institutional Review Boards (IRBs) to review and approve research

---

[23] Torbay, J. (2023). The work of Donald Ewen Cameron: from psychic driving to MK Ultra. *History of Psychiatry.* 34(3):320–330. doi: 10.1177/0957154X231163763.

[24] Academic (2022) Donald Ewen Cameron. Available at https://en-academic.com/dic.nsf/enwiki/462457 (Accessed 2/13/24).

involving human subjects, ensuring that ethical standards are upheld. The legacy of Cameron's work serves as a reminder of the potential for abuse in medical research and the critical importance of ethical guidelines to protect participants in scientific studies.

Sanctions

Despite the significant ethical violations and harm caused by his experiments, Dr. Cameron was never formally sanctioned or held legally accountable for his actions during his lifetime. The lack of immediate accountability can be attributed to several factors, including the era's limited awareness and enforcement of research ethics, the covert nature of the funding and support his experiments received from the CIA as part of MK-Ultra, and the general lack of regulatory frameworks at the time to address such abuses in medical research.

The revelations about Cameron's experiments and their impact on patients came to light years after they were conducted, primarily through investigative journalism and the efforts of former patients and their families seeking justice and recognition of their suffering. While these revelations led to public outrage and contributed to significant changes in the ethical oversight of research involving human subjects, Cameron himself did not face direct consequences in terms of legal or professional sanctions.

Dr. Cameron passed away in 1967 from a heart attack while mountain climbing. He died before the full extent of the ethical breaches and the harm caused by his experiments was widely known or acknowledged. It was only in the years following his death, particularly during the 1970s and 1980s with the Church Committee investigations and subsequent inquiries into MK-Ultra, that the unethical nature of his work was fully exposed.

The absence of sanctions against Cameron highlights the historical gaps in ethical oversight and accountability in medical research, underscoring the importance of the reforms and safeguards that have since been established to protect participants in scientific studies. These include the requirement for informed consent, the establishment of Institutional Review Boards (IRBs), and the development of ethical guidelines such as the Belmont Report, which emphasize respect for persons, beneficence, and justice in research.

Conclusion

The Montreal Experiments, spearheaded by Dr. Donald Ewen Cameron at the Allan Memorial Institute, stand as a vivid reminder of the ethical boundaries that were crossed in the pursuit of understanding and controlling the human mind. Despite the initial intent to advance psychiatric treatment, the experiments resulted in profound and lasting harm to many individuals, undermining the very essence of medical ethics and human dignity. The legacy of these experiments has not only shed light on the dark chapters of psychiatric research but also catalyzed significant reforms in research ethics, emphasizing the paramount importance of informed consent, the welfare of participants, and the ethical responsibilities of researchers. As we reflect on the Montreal Experiments, it becomes evident that the pursuit of scientific knowledge must never compromise the fundamental rights and well-being of individuals, ensuring that such ethical transgressions are never repeated in the annals of medical research.

Further Reading

1. **"In the Sleep Room: The Story of the CIA Brainwashing Experiments in Canada" by Ann Collins, January 1, 1998, Key Porter Books**
   - This book provides a detailed and disturbing account of Dr. Ewen Cameron's CIA-sponsored psychic-torture experiments during the Cold War era, focusing on the impact on patients.

Chapter 9

Henrietta Lacks: The Legacy of Immortality and Injustice

Henrietta Lacks' (Figure 1) story is one of the most ethically challenging and fascinating in medical history. Born Loretta Pleasant on August 1, 1920, in Roanoke, Virginia, Henrietta experienced hardship early on.[1] She grew up in a log cabin that once housed slaves in Clover, Virginia, and was raised by her grandfather after her mother died in 1924. In 1941, she married David "Day" Lacks and moved to Turner Station, Maryland, for a better life. They had five children, but her life was cut short by cervical cancer at 31.

In 1951, while seeking treatment at Johns Hopkins Hospital, doctors took a biopsy of her cancer without her consent. This led to the creation of the HeLa cell line, the first immortal human cell line, which has been crucial for medical research.[2] Henrietta died and was buried in an unmarked grave, her contribution unknown for decades.

Henrietta's story highlights significant ethical issues in medical research, including consent, privacy, and individual rights. Despite the lack of consent, her HeLa cells have led to major medical breakthroughs. Recently, her contributions have been acknowledged, including a research

---

[1] https://msa.maryland.gov/msa/educ/exhibits/womenshallfame/html/lacks.html#:~:text=
Henrietta%20Lacks%2C%20born%20as%20Loretta,%2C%20on%20April%2010%2C%
201941 (Accessed 2/15/24).

[2] Stump, J.L. (2014). Henrietta Lacks and the HeLa cell: Rights of patients and responsibilities of medical researchers. *The History Teacher*. 48(1):127–180.

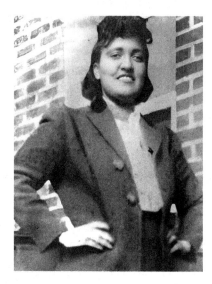

Figure 1.   Henrietta Lacks.
Source: Wikimedia Commons.

building named in her honor at Johns Hopkins University. Her legacy continues to prompt discussions on scientific ethics and the need for reforms to protect individuals' rights. This chapter explores Henrietta's life, her lasting impact, and the ethical questions her story raises.

The Discovery of HeLa Cells

Dr. George Otto Gey,[3] a prominent researcher at Johns Hopkins, was the scientist who received Henrietta's cells. At the time, the practice of using patient samples for research without explicit consent was commonplace and legally permissible. Henrietta's cells, taken during a routine biopsy, were cultured by Dr. Gey to create an immortal cell line — a line of cells that could reproduce indefinitely in the lab if the fundamental cell survival conditions were met. This was a feat that had never been accomplished with human cells.

---

[3] https://embryo.asu.edu/pages/george-otto-gey-1899-1970 (Accessed 2/13/24).

Before the advent of HeLa cells, cell culture in medical research faced significant challenges that limited the scope and duration of scientific studies. Traditional human cell cultures would only survive for a few days outside the body, making it difficult to conduct long-term experiments or to observe the effects of treatments over extended periods.[4] This short lifespan of cultured cells hindered the progress in understanding complex biological processes and in testing the efficacy and safety of potential new treatments. Moreover, the variability between cell samples from different individuals introduced inconsistencies that complicated the replication of experiments and the interpretation of results.

The introduction of HeLa cells represented a monumental shift in the field of cell biology and medical research. Their unique properties addressed many of the problems associated with earlier cell cultures:

- **Immortality**: HeLa cells were the first human cells found to be "immortal" in the laboratory, meaning they could divide an unlimited number of times if provided with the right conditions. This immortality allowed for continuous experimentation and observation over much longer periods than was previously possible, opening new avenues for research into the fundamental mechanisms of life, disease progression, and the long-term effects of drugs.
- **Durability and Rapid Reproduction**: HeLa cells were not only durable, and capable of surviving and thriving under conditions that would be challenging for other cell types, but they also reproduced at an unprecedented rate. HeLa cells can double their cell count in 24 hrs.[5] This rapid reproduction facilitated the production of large quantities of uniform cells, essential for experiments requiring significant amounts of biological material. The robust nature of HeLa cells

---

[4] Ulrich, A.B. and Pour, P.M. (2001). *Encyclopedia of Genetics.*
[5] https://www.tebubio.com/blog/hela-cells-the-first-cell-line/#:~:text=2%2D%20HeLa%20cells%20grow%20unusually,and%20overtake%20other%20cell%20cultures.

reduced the variability seen with primary cell cultures and allowed for more consistent and reliable experimental results.

- **Enabling Previously Impossible Research**: The properties of HeLa cells allowed scientists to undertake research that was previously impossible. For example, they provided a stable, consistent model for studying the effects of viruses on human cells, leading to significant advancements in virology. The development of the polio vaccine by Jonas Salk is a prime example of how HeLa cells enabled ground-breaking research. The cells were used to grow poliovirus in large quantities, which was crucial for testing the vaccine's efficacy and safety before it was administered to humans. Furthermore, HeLa cells have been instrumental in genetic research, including the study of chromosomes and gene expression, paving the way for advancements in genetic engineering and the understanding of genetic diseases.

- **Facilitating Drug Testing and Development**: The consistent and replicable nature of HeLa cells provided an ideal platform for drug testing and development. Researchers could observe the effects of drugs on a standardized human cell line over extended periods, significantly improving the process of evaluating drug toxicity, mechanisms of action, and potential side effects. This has been particularly important in cancer research, where HeLa cells have been used to test the efficacy of chemotherapy agents and to explore new treatment strategies.

HeLa cells overcame the limitations of previous cell culture methods, offering a durable, immortal, and rapidly reproducing cell line that has become a cornerstone of modern medical research. Their introduction has not only revolutionized the field of cell biology but also facilitated countless scientific breakthroughs, contributing to our understanding of disease and the development of new therapies.

The impact of HeLa cells on medical science cannot be overstated. They have been instrumental in numerous scientific breakthroughs and medical advancements:

- **Polio Vaccine**: HeLa cells played a crucial role in the development of the polio vaccine by Jonas Salk in the 1950s. The cells provided a reliable medium for testing the vaccine, ultimately leading to its widespread distribution and the near-eradication of polio.[6,7,8]

- **Cancer Research**: HeLa cells have been used extensively in cancer research, contributing to our understanding of cancer cell biology, the effects of radiation and chemotherapy, and the development of new treatments.[9,10]
- **COVID-19 Vaccines**: More recently, HeLa cells have been used in research to combat the COVID-19 pandemic, including the development and testing of vaccines.[11] Their use has accelerated the pace of COVID-19 research, demonstrating the enduring value of HeLa cells in addressing emergent global health crises.
- **Effects of Radiation on Cells**: HeLa cells were placed in the Russian Mir space station for 40 days and in the American space shuttle for 9 days to study the ability of space radiation to cause breaks in DNA strands.[12]

---

[6] Turner, T. (2012) Development of the polio vaccine: a historical perspective of Tuskegee University's role in mass production and distribution of HeLa cells. *J Health Care Poor Underserved*. 23(4 Suppl):5–10. doi: 10.1353/hpu.2012.0151.

[7] Salk, J. (1955). Use of HeLa cell culture for the production and control of polio vaccine. *Journal of Immunology*.

[8] Scherer, W.F., Syverton, J.T. and Gey, G.O. (1953). Studies on the propagation *in vitro* of poliomyelitis viruses. IV. Viral multiplication in a stable strain of human malignant epithelial cells (strain HeLa) derived from an epidermoid carcinoma of the cervix. *J Exp Med*. 97(5):695–710. doi: 10.1084/jem.97.5.695. PMID: 13052828; PMCID: PMC2136303.

[9] Lengauer, C., Kinzler, K. and Vogelstein, B. (1998). Genetic instabilities in human cancers. *Nature* 396: 643–649. https://doi.org/10.1038/25292.

[10] Puck, T.T., Marcus, P.I. and Cieciura, S.J. (1956). Clonal growth of mammalian cells in vitro; growth characteristics of colonies from single HeLa cells with and without a feeder layer. *J Exp Med*. 103(2):273–83. doi: 10.1084/jem.103.2.273.

[11] Zhou, P., Yang, XL. and Wang, XG. *et al.* (2020). A pneumonia outbreak associated with a new coronavirus of probable bat origin. *Nature* 579:270–273. https://doi.org/10.1038/s41586-020-2012-7.

[12] Takeo, O., Ken, O., Akihisa, T., Yoshitaka, T., Masaru, S., Tamotsu, N. and Shunji, N. (2002). Detection of DNA Damage Induced by Space Radiation in Mir and Space Shuttle. *Journal of Radiation Research*, 43(Suppl): Pages S133–S136, https://doi.org/10.1269/jrr.43.S133.

Ethical Violations and Consent

Human tissue samples are key to medical and scientific breakthroughs, especially in the push toward personalized medicine.[13] Research using these samples has led to major discoveries about human health, including new ways to diagnose, treat, and prevent diseases. In cancer research, the use of tissue samples has grown significantly, shedding light on the molecular causes of cancer, and leading to new methods for assessing risk, diagnosing conditions, and developing treatments.[14]

However, the use of human tissue samples in research brings up important issues. These include how informed consent is obtained, how research is overseen, how data is shared on a large scale, and how privacy and confidentiality are protected. Other concerns include the commercial use of samples, how research findings are accessed, and the rights of individuals to withdraw from research.[15] Successfully navigating these issues is crucial. It requires approaches that the public and patients find acceptable, and it depends on building and maintaining their support, trust, and transparency.

Informed Consent

It is helpful here to briefly discuss the topic of informed consent. The purpose of informed consent is multifaceted, serving legal, ethical, and administrative functions in medical practice. Legally, it originated from the principle established in 1914 that a patient has the right to decide what happens to his body,[16] evolving over time to require physicians to disclose information that a reasonable person would want to know for making

---

[13] Bledsoe, M.J. and Grizzle, W.E. (2013). Use of human specimens in research: the evolving United States regulatory, policy, and scientific landscape. *Diagn. Histopathol.* 19:322–330.

[14] Hughes, S.E., Barnes, R.O. and Watson, P.H. (2010). Biospecimen use in cancer research over two decades. *Biopreserv. Biobank.* 8:89–97.

[15] McGuire, A.L. and Beskow, L.M. (2010). Informed consent in genomics and genetic research. *Annu. Rev. Genom. Hum. Genet.* 11:361–381.

[16] Schloendorff, V. *Society of New York Hospital.* Vol. 211 N.Y. 125, 105 N.E. 921914.

informed decisions about his treatment.[17] This legal aspect protects patients against unwanted medical interventions (i.e., assault and battery) and upholds their rights to autonomy and self-determination. Ethically, informed consent respects patient autonomy by ensuring that medical or surgical treatments align with the patient's desires and choices, emphasizing that it is a continuous process rather than a one-time event. Administratively, informed consent documents serve as a system-level check to confirm that the consent process has occurred, although this can sometimes reduce the process of obtaining a signature under pressure for efficiency. Current medical practice requires that medical professionals first assess the patient's capacity to understand the elements of informed consent. Having satisfied themselves that the patient is competent to make health care decisions, they must discuss the following topics with the patient before seeking to obtain informed consent: the diagnosis, the proposed treatment, the risks and benefits associated with the treatment, as well as the risks and benefits associated with declining the treatment. To conform with the Joint Commission regulations,[18] the provider must document all the elements of informed consent in the medical record.[19] It should be noted that informed consent is not only required for medical and surgical treatments but for the dissemination of patient information.

The story of Henrietta Lacks and the removal of HeLa cells from her cervical cancer tissue without her knowledge or consent highlight a significant ethical violation of that trust and transparency in the annals of medical research. At the time, the prevailing medical and legal standards did not require doctors to obtain consent from patients for the use of their tissues in research.[20]

---

[17] Berg, J.W. Appelbaum, P. and Lidz, C. *et al.* (2001). The Legal Requirements for Disclosure and Consent: History and Current Status. In: *Informed Consent: Legal Theory and Clinical Practice.* 2nd ed New York (NY): Oxford University Press. p. 41–74.

[18] Standards–The Joint Commission (RC.02.01.01, RI.01.03.01, RI.01.03.03, RI.01.03.05).

[19] Slim, K. and Bazin, J.E. (2019). From informed consent to shared decision-making in surgery. *J Visc Surg.* 156(3):181–184.

[20] Smith, V. (April 17 2002). Wonder Woman: The Life, Death, and Life After Death of Henrietta Lacks, Unwitting Heroine of Modern Medical Science. *Baltimore City Paper.*

Legality

Today, the research use of patient tissue acquired during treatment remains legal. For example, in the 1990 case of Moore v. Regents of the University of California,[21] the California Supreme Court decided that once a patient's tissue samples are taken for research, the patient no longer owns those samples. This means that the tissue and cells can be used for commercial purposes without the person's ownership claim.[22] The justices in this case worried that giving patients property rights over their tissues would "hinder research by restricting access to the necessary raw materials" and might "destroy the economic incentive to conduct important medical research." Since this decision, many U.S. courts have ruled against family members who have taken legal action against researchers and universities for using their deceased relative's body parts for commercial purposes without permission.[23]

The Ethical Transformation in Medical Research: The Legacy of Henrietta Lacks

Henrietta Lacks' story has been pivotal in evolving the ethical standards in medical research, particularly around informed consent. In the 1950s, the concept of informed consent was nebulous, with the Nuremberg Code of 1947[24] — established post-Nuremberg Trials — being inconsistently applied, especially in the use of patient tissues for research. Henrietta Lacks' case, where her cells were used without consent to create the HeLa cell line, exemplifies the ethical lapses of the time.

Since then, the ethical landscape has undergone significant reform. Modern guidelines, including the National Research Act,[25] Belmont

---

[21] *John Moore, Plaintiff and Appellant, v. The Regents of the University of California et al., Defendants and Respondents.* 793 P.2d 479, 51 Cal. 3d 120, 271 Cal. Rptr. 146

[22] Sandra B. (July 10, 1990). Patient's Right to Tissue Is Limited. *New York Times.*

[23] Epstein, R.A. Sharkey, C (2016). *Cases and Materials on Torts.* Aspen Casebook Series (11th ed.). New York: Wolters Kluwer. p. 560.

[24] Moreno, J.D., Schmidt. U. and Joffe, S. The Nuremberg Code 70 Years Later. *JAMA.* 318(9):795–796. doi: 10.1001/jama.2017.10265.

[25] https://www.congress.gov/bill/93rd-congress/house-bill/7724 (Accessed 2/27/24).

Report,[26] and various national regulations, now underscore the importance of informed consent, respect for persons, beneficence, and justice. These guidelines mandate that researchers obtain informed consent, detailing the research's purpose, procedures, risks, and benefits. Additionally, the use of human tissues in research must undergo ethical review to protect participants' rights. They have spurred significant debate and policy changes regarding the use of human biological materials, patient consent, and the sharing of benefits arising from research.[27] The National Institutes of Health (NIH) agreement with the Lacks family in 2013, granting them some control over the use of HeLa cells' genomic data,[28] reflects an evolving recognition of the need to address ethical issues retrospectively and to honor the contributions of research participants.

Lacks' influence extends globally, impacting international ethical standards such as the Declaration of Helsinki[29] and the guidelines by the Council for International Organizations of Medical Sciences (CIOMS),[30] which reflect a consensus on the importance of consent and ethical use of human biological materials. These developments underscore the global resonance of Lacks' story in shaping ethical discourse.

Despite these advancements, Lacks' legacy continues to fuel debates on the adequacy of current ethical standards and the balance between scientific progress and individual rights. Her story highlights the ongoing disparities in medical research, particularly affecting minority and economically disadvantaged populations. This aspect of her legacy calls for a reflection on ethical standards and the importance of ensuring dignity, respect, and fairness.

---

[26] https://www.hhs.gov/ohrp/regulations-and-policy/belmont-report/index.html (Accessed 2/27/24).

[27] Hudson, K.L. and Collins, F.S. (2013). Biospecimen policy: family matters. *Nature.* 500:141–142.

[28] https://www.nih.gov/news-events/news-releases/nih-lacks-family-reach-understanding-share-genomic-data-hela-cells (Accessed 2/15/24).

[29] https://www.wma.net/policies-post/wma-declaration-of-helsinki-ethical-principles-for-medical-research-involving-human-subjects/ (Accessed 2/27/24).

[30] https://cioms.ch/ (Accessed 2/15/24).

Regulatory Impact

Henrietta Lacks' case has significantly influenced U.S. federal guidelines on informed consent, particularly through the Common Rule's adoption and subsequent revisions. The Common Rule,[31] so named because it was adopted in 1991 by 15 federal departments and agencies simultaneously, is officially known as Subpart A of the Health and Human Services (HHS) regulations (45CFR46). It establishes comprehensive protections for research subjects, emphasizing informed consent and ethical standards in research involving human subjects.

The HHS regulations include three additional subparts (B, C, & D) beyond the Common Rule, offering extra protections for vulnerable research participant groups. The revisions to the Common Rule, inspired by the Lacks case, have expanded these protections to cover biological specimens. This change underscores a significant shift toward valuing individual autonomy in decisions about the use of personal biological materials, a principle notably absent in Henrietta Lacks' experience.

Conclusion

The story of Henrietta Lacks encapsulated in the development of HeLa cell cultures demonstrates the profound impact one individual's life can have on science and ethics. Henrietta's legacy is not merely one of scientific immortality but also a narrative that underscores the critical importance of ethical considerations in medical research. Her story serves as a vital example of the need to balance scientific advancement with the respect and protection of individual rights.

Henrietta Lacks' contributions to science, though made without her consent, have facilitated countless medical breakthroughs and advancements. The HeLa cell line has been instrumental in developing vaccines, understanding cancer, and even combating global pandemics like

---

[31] https://www.hhs.gov/ohrp/education-and-outreach/about-research-participation/protecting-research-volunteers/principal-regulations/index.html#:~:text=The%20Common%20Rule%20generally%20requires,in%20language%20they%20would%20understand (Accessed 2/37/24).

COVID-19. However, how her cells were obtained and used without acknowledgment or compensation for decades highlights significant ethical oversights that cannot be ignored.

The legacy of Henrietta Lacks has catalyzed a much-needed discourse on consent, privacy, and the rights of individuals in medical research. It has prompted a reevaluation of ethical standards, leading to more stringent guidelines for obtaining informed consent and ensuring the dignity and rights of research participants are upheld. The establishment of The Henrietta Lacks Foundation and the recognition of her contributions by the scientific community are steps toward rectifying past injustices. Yet, they also remind us of the ongoing need for vigilance and commitment to ethical practices in research.

Moreover, Henrietta's story sheds light on the racial and socio-economic disparities that persist in medical research, calling for a more equitable approach that respects and protects all individuals, regardless of their background. It is a stark reminder that the benefits of scientific research should not come at the expense of individual rights and dignity.

The legacy of Henrietta Lacks compels us to continuously evaluate and improve the ethical standards governing medical research. It is a call to action for researchers, ethicists, and policymakers alike to ensure that scientific advancement progresses hand in hand with respect for the rights and contributions of individuals. Henrietta Lacks' story, marked by both immortality and injustice, serves as a powerful reminder of the human element at the heart of scientific discovery. It underscores the imperative to balance the pursuit of knowledge with the ethical obligations we owe to those who contribute, knowingly or unknowingly, to the advancement of medicine. As we move forward, let Henrietta Lacks' legacy guide us toward a future where scientific progress is achieved with integrity, respect, and a commitment to ethical principles.

Further Reading

The most notable book written about Henrietta Lacks is *The Immortal Life of Henrietta Lacks* by Rebecca Skloot. Published in 2010, this non-fiction work delves into the life, death, and enduring legacy of Henrietta Lacks, whose cells (HeLa cells) were taken without her consent and became one of the most important tools in medicine. Skloot's book explores the collision between ethics, race, and medicine; it highlights the scientific discovery and faith healing, and the deep injustice experienced by the Lacks family. The book has received critical acclaim for its thorough research, engaging narrative, and exploration of the complex ethical issues surrounding medical research and consent. It was the 2011 winner of the National Academies Communication Award for best creative work that helps the public understand topics in science, engineering, or medicine.

Chapter 10

The SUPPORT Study Controversy: Ethics, Premature Infants, and Parental Consent

The Surfactant, Positive Pressure, and Oxygenation Randomized Trial (SUPPORT) study,[1] conducted from 2005 to 2009, represents a pivotal moment in the intersection of neonatal care, medical research, and bioethics. This ambitious clinical trial aimed to determine the optimal oxygen saturation levels in extremely premature infants (see Figure 1) to minimize the risk of retinopathy of prematurity (ROP) without increasing other adverse outcomes, such as death or neurodevelopmental disabilities. The study's significance lies not only in its potential to refine treatment protocols and improve outcomes for one of the most vulnerable patient populations but also in the ethical challenges it presented, particularly regarding informed consent.

The controversy surrounding the SUPPORT study centers on the ethical considerations involved in conducting research on premature infants and the adequacy of the informed consent process. In essence, the researchers needed to tell the parents that if their child was put into the study, the child would be randomly placed in one of two groups. In the "low oxygen" group, the likelihood of death or severe neurological disability was increased. In the "high oxygen" group, the likelihood of blindness was increased. These risks were not communicated to the parents.

---

[1] https://classic.clinicaltrials.gov/ct2/show/NCT00233324 (Accessed 2/25/24).

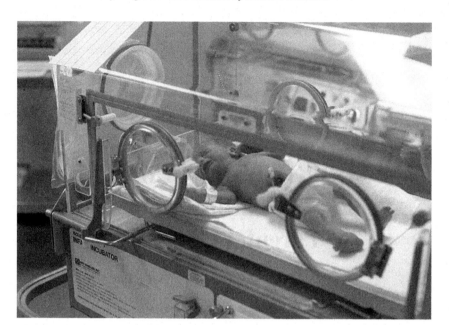

Figure 1.   Neonate in an incubator.

As a result, critics argue that the consent forms used in the study failed to adequately disclose the risks associated with participation, including the increased risk of death or severe retinopathy in certain oxygen saturation target groups. This omission raised profound ethical concerns, highlighting the tension between the pursuit of scientific knowledge and the imperative to protect research subjects, especially when those subjects are incapable of advocating for themselves.

The ethical debate surrounding the SUPPORT study underscores the critical importance of informed consent in medical research. Informed consent is not merely a procedural formality but a fundamental patient right and a cornerstone of ethical research practice. The controversy reveals the complexities of obtaining truly informed consent in neonatal research, where parents must make decisions on behalf of their critically ill infants under conditions of uncertainty and emotional distress.

This chapter explores the SUPPORT study controversy in depth, examining the ethical dilemmas it raises and the lessons it offers for future research involving vulnerable populations. By dissecting the intricacies of this case, we aim to shed light on the delicate balance between advancing medical science and upholding the highest ethical standards in research.

Understanding the SUPPORT Study

The history of oxygen use in neonatology highlights a complex journey marked by both advancements and setbacks. Initially recommended in the early 1900s for premature infants experiencing cyanosis, oxygen was used liberally in incubators without concrete evidence of its benefits. This practice led to the unintended consequence of retrolental fibroplasia, a form of blindness. Stevie Wonder's blindness is a result of this phenomenon. The realization in the 1950s that excessive oxygen contributed to this condition prompted restrictions on its use, which then resulted in increased rates of death and cerebral palsy among infants. Subsequent analysis suggested a stark trade-off: for every infant saved from blindness, 16 others died.

Advancements in neonatology, including the discovery of surfactants, the use of antenatal corticosteroids, improved nutrition, gentler ventilators, and specialized care in intensive care units, have significantly enhanced the survival rates of extremely premature infants. Despite these improvements, the following question still existed: "What is the optimal oxygen saturation level for extremely premature infants that balances the reduction of retinopathy of prematurity (ROP) risk with the maximization of survival rates?" The Surfactant, Positive Pressure, and Oxygenation Randomized Trial (SUPPORT) was a landmark clinical trial designed to address this critical question. This section delves into the study's goals, design, participant selection process, and methodology, providing a comprehensive understanding of its scope and significance.

The primary goal of the SUPPORT study was to determine the most beneficial oxygen saturation levels for premature infants to minimize the risk of ROP, a potentially blinding condition, while also ensuring the highest possible survival rates without increasing the risk of other serious outcomes like neurological damage. ROP is a disease state characterized by abnormal blood vessel growth in the retina, primarily affecting infants born before 31 weeks of gestation. The condition can lead to vision impairment and blindness, making its prevention a priority in neonatal care. However, the administration of oxygen, a vital treatment for premature infants with underdeveloped lungs, needed careful optimization to avoid exacerbating the risk of ROP while supporting overall health and development.[2]

The SUPPORT study was a multicenter, randomized controlled trial that enrolled 1,316 extremely preterm infants born between 24 and 27 weeks of gestation from 2005 to 2009. The study was meticulously designed to compare two target ranges of oxygen saturation: a lower range (85–89%) and a higher range (91–95%). These ranges were chosen based on prior research suggesting that lower oxygen levels might reduce the risk of ROP, but concerns remained about whether such levels could negatively impact survival and lead to other complications.

Participants were randomly assigned to one of the two oxygen saturation target groups immediately after birth. Specialized pulse oximeters, modified to display oxygen saturation levels within a 3% range of the actual values, were used to maintain the assigned oxygen saturation targets without revealing the exact levels to the clinical staff. This blinding was crucial to prevent bias in the administration of supplemental oxygen and ensure the reliability of the study's findings.

The methodology employed in the SUPPORT study was groundbreaking in its attempt to clarify the optimal management of oxygen therapy in premature infants. By comparing the outcomes of infants in the two target ranges, researchers hoped to provide definitive guidance on oxygen saturation levels that could improve survival rates while minimizing the risk of ROP and other oxygen-related complications.

Clinical Results

The results of the SUPPORT study, published in *The New England Journal of Medicine* in 2010, revealed complex outcomes.[3] Infants in the

---

[2] Tin, W., Milligan, D.W., Pennefather, P. and Hey, E. (Mar 2001) Pulse oximetry, severe retinopathy, and outcome at one year in babies of less than 28 weeks gestation. *Arch Dis Child Fetal Neonatal Ed.* 84(2):F106–F110. doi: 10.1136/fn.84.2.f106.

[3] SUPPORT Study Group of the Eunice Kennedy Shriver NICHD Neonatal Research Network. Target Ranges of Oxygen Saturation in Extremely Preterm Infants, May 27, 2010, *N Engl J Med* 2010; 362:1959–1969. doi: 10.1056/NEJMoa0911781.

lower oxygen saturation target group had a reduced risk of ROP. However, this group also experienced a higher mortality rate compared to the higher oxygen saturation target group. Conversely, infants in the higher oxygen saturation target group had a higher risk of ROP but a lower mortality rate. These findings highlighted the delicate balance between reducing the risk of severe ROP and the risk of mortality in extremely premature infants, underscoring the challenges in managing oxygen therapy in neonatal care.

The SUPPORT study's results have had a profound impact on clinical practice and guidelines for the care of premature infants, prompting ongoing discussions and further research into the best approaches for oxygen management in this vulnerable population.

The Ethical Dilemma: Informed Consent and Risk Disclosure in the SUPPORT Study

The Surfactant, Positive Pressure, and Oxygenation Randomized Trial (SUPPORT) study, while aiming to address critical questions in neonatal care, became embroiled in an ethical controversy centered around the informed consent process. This section examines the informed consent procedure utilized in the SUPPORT study, discusses the allegations of inadequate risk disclosure to the parents of participating infants, and analyzes the ethical standards for informed consent, especially concerning vulnerable populations like premature infants.

The informed consent process for the study has come under scrutiny for allegedly failing to fully disclose the risks involved, including the potential for death or severe disability. Informed consent in clinical research is predicated on the principle of autonomy, requiring that participants or their surrogates are fully informed about the nature of the study, its purpose, potential benefits, and risks before agreeing to participate.[4]

---

[4] Lorell, B.H., Mikita, J.S., Anderson, A., Hallinan, Z.P. and Forrest, A. (2015) Informed consent in clinical research: Consensus recommendations for reform identified by an expert interview panel. *Clin Trials.* 12(6):692–695. doi: 10.1177/1740774515594362. Epub 2015 Jul 15.

Critics of the SUPPORT study contend that the consent forms provided to the parents did not adequately communicate the risks associated with the different oxygen saturation levels being tested. Specifically, concerns were raised that parents were not clearly informed that being in one of the study's arms could potentially increase the risk of death or lead to severe disabilities compared to standard care practices outside the study framework. The Office for Human Research Protections (OHRP), the group responsible for protecting the rights and welfare of human subjects involved in research conducted or supported by the US Department of Health and Human Services (HHS), criticized the study's consent forms for this lack of clarity.[5]

The OHRP and other critics[6] reported the consent forms had many deficiencies. These deficiencies primarily revolve around the failure to adequately inform participants — or, in this case, the parents of the infant participants — about the nature of the research, the risks involved, and the experimental nature of certain procedures. This critique is grounded in the principles outlined in the U.S. Code of Federal Regulations[7] which stipulates the requirements for informed consent in research. The SUPPORT study's consent forms were found lacking in several key areas:

The consent forms did not sufficiently explain that the study involved research with experimental aspects. An essential requirement of informed consent is to inform participants that the study is research, outlining its purposes clearly. This omission undermines the ability of parents to understand that their infants were being enrolled in a study that sought to test hypotheses rather than provide established care.

The consent forms failed to convey the full spectrum of risks. For example, none of the consent forms explicitly mentioned death as a potential risk of the oxygen interventions being studied nor did they adequately explain that the higher levels could lead to an increased risk of severe retinopathy of prematurity (ROP), a condition that can result in blindness

---

[5] Department of Health and Human Services, Office for Human Research Protections. Letter to the University of Alabama at Birmingham. March 7, 2013 (http://www.hhs.gov/ohrp/detrm_letrs/YR13/mar13a.pdf. opens in new tab) (Accessed 2/15/24).

[6] Wilfond, B.S, *et al.* (2013). The OHRP and SUPPORT. *N Engl J Med.* 368(25):e36. doi: 10.1056/NEJMc1307008. Epub 2013 Jun 5.

[7] 45CFR46.116.

(see footnote 6). This is a critical omission, given that the study aimed to explore the optimal oxygen saturation levels for extremely premature infants, a population already at high risk for mortality and severe morbidity. The forms also failed to provide a comprehensive description of reasonably foreseeable risks or discomforts, which is a fundamental aspect of enabling informed decision-making.

The use of modified oximeters to mask the infants' oxygen-saturation levels was a key experimental component of the SUPPORT study. However, this was not adequately disclosed in the consent forms. Understanding that certain procedures are experimental is crucial for parents to make informed decisions about their infants' participation in research.

The consent forms lacked sufficient information on alternative courses of treatment that might have been advantageous to the subjects. This information is vital for participants or their surrogates to weigh the benefits and risks of study participation against those associated with other available treatments.

Approximately half of the consent forms suggested that all treatments proposed in the study were standard of care, implying no expected increase in risk. This representation was misleading because the study's design — to hold oxygen levels at either end of a wide range considered safe — differed from usual clinical care. It obscured the fact that the potential risks and benefits of study participation were not equivalent to those of receiving care outside the study's structured protocol.

The SUPPORT study's consent process failed to meet the ethical and regulatory standards for informed consent, particularly in the context of research involving vulnerable populations such as premature infants. The deficiencies in the consent forms compromised the ability of parents to make fully informed decisions about their infants' participation, highlighting a significant ethical lapse in the study's execution. The OHRP's determination in March 2013 underscored the seriousness of these deficiencies, emphasizing the need for rigorous adherence to informed consent standards in all research involving human subjects.

The OHRP highlighted the ethical imperative to ensure that participants or their surrogates can make informed decisions based on a comprehensive understanding of the risks involved.

The ethical standards for informed consent are particularly stringent when it comes to vulnerable populations, such as premature infants. These standards are grounded in the principles of beneficence, to do good; non-maleficence, to do no harm; and respect for persons, which includes respecting their autonomy and protecting those with diminished autonomy. The American Academy of Pediatrics (AAP) and other bodies have emphasized the need for heightened protections when obtaining consent from parents or guardians of neonates for participation in research. This includes ensuring that the information provided is clear, comprehensive, and communicated in a manner that is understandable to non-medical professionals.

The Fallout: Public and Professional Response

The revelations concerning the informed consent process in the Surfactant, Positive Pressure, and Oxygenation Randomized Trial (SUPPORT) study catalyzed a wide range of responses from the public, academic circles, bioethicists, pediatricians, and advocacy groups. These reactions were varied, reflecting a spectrum of opinions on the ethical considerations of conducting clinical research on vulnerable populations, such as premature infants.

The academic response was swift and multifaceted, with numerous articles and commentaries published in medical and ethics journals. Scholars and clinicians debated the ethical implications of the SUPPORT study, particularly focusing on the adequacy of the informed consent process. For instance, an article in *The New England Journal of Medicine* by Hudson, Guttmacher, and Collins from the National Institutes of Health (NIH) defended the study's intentions and its adherence to ethical standards, arguing that the controversy highlighted the challenges of communicating complex research risks and benefits to participants.[8] Conversely, a group of bioethicists and neonatologists published a critique in the same journal, emphasizing the need for clearer risk communication in consent forms (see footnote 5).

---

[8] Hudson, K.L., Guttmacher, A.E. and Collins, F.S. (2013) Support of SUPPORT — A View from the NIH. *N Engl J Med.* 368:2349–2351.

Bioethicists played a crucial role in dissecting the ethical nuances of the SUPPORT study, with many expressing concerns over the potential underestimation and undercommunication of risks involved in the study. The debate extended beyond the specifics of the SUPPORT study to broader discussions about the ethics of clinical research involving children and the necessity of rigorous informed consent processes. These discussions often highlighted the tension between advancing medical knowledge and ensuring the protection and autonomy of research subjects.

Pediatricians and neonatologists, particularly those working directly with premature infants and their families, expressed a range of reactions. Some defended the study as a necessary step toward improving outcomes for premature infants, while others criticized it for ethical lapses in the consent process. The AAP issued statements emphasizing the importance of ethical standards in neonatal research and the need for transparency and clarity in the informed consent process.

Advocacy groups, especially those representing families of premature infants, voiced strong concerns about the SUPPORT study. These groups demanded greater accountability and transparency in medical research, calling for reforms to ensure that parents are fully informed about the risks and benefits of research participation. Their responses highlighted the emotional and ethical weight of decision-making for parents of vulnerable infants and the imperative of trust in the physician-researcher relationship.

The media played a pivotal role in shaping public perception of the SUPPORT study, with coverage ranging from investigative reports to opinion pieces in major newspapers and online platforms. The media's involvement brought the debate to a wider audience, raising awareness about the complexities of medical research ethics and the specific challenges of conducting research with premature infants. Coverage in the media also amplified the voices of concerned parents and advocacy groups, contributing to a broader public discourse on the ethical obligations of researchers to their subjects.

The fallout from the SUPPORT study's consent controversy thus spanned multiple spheres, from academic journals to public forums, reflecting a diverse array of perspectives on the ethical challenges of neonatal research. The discussions it prompted have had lasting implications for the field of medical ethics, particularly regarding informed consent and the conduct of research involving vulnerable populations.

Regulatory and Institutional Scrutiny

The SUPPORT trial, which sought to refine oxygen therapy protocols for premature infants, faced intense scrutiny from regulatory and institutional bodies due to concerns over its informed consent process. The Office for OHRP, tasked with safeguarding the rights and welfare of research subjects, conducted an in-depth review of the study's consent procedures. The findings were stark, revealing that the consent documents did not fully communicate the risks involved in the study, notably the potential for death or significant disability stemming from the different oxygen levels used. This deficiency in risk disclosure raised profound ethical issues, potentially impairing the capacity of parents to make truly informed decisions regarding their infants' involvement in the study.

In reaction to the OHRP's critique, the National Institutes of Health (NIH), the study's financier, undertook measures to address the raised concerns. A pivotal initiative was the launch of a comprehensive dialogue on the ethical and regulatory hurdles presented by comparative effectiveness research, with a particular focus on studies involving vulnerable groups, such as premature infants. The NIH recognized the inherent challenges in adequately informing participants about the risks and benefits of studies that compare interventions already deemed standard of care but lacking in direct comparative analysis for effectiveness and safety.

Moreover, the NIH pledged to formulate more explicit guidelines for informed consent in these research scenarios, aiming to bolster the transparency and depth of information relayed to research participants or their proxies. This effort sought to better elucidate the risks tied to participation and the investigational nature of certain study interventions.

The fallout from the SUPPORT trial also spurred a reevaluation of research practices and consent protocols among the participating institutions. Numerous academic and research entities involved in the trial scrutinized their informed consent processes, especially those concerning research with vulnerable populations. This introspection led to an enhanced recognition of the necessity for clear communication of risks and the ethical obligation to guarantee that participants, or their guardians, are thoroughly briefed on the research's potential impacts.

The scrutiny faced by the SUPPORT trial has left a durable mark on clinical research, especially within neonatology. It highlighted the imperative for stringent ethical standards in trial design and execution, the necessity for transparent and effective risk and benefit communication, and the continuous duty of research bodies to safeguard participant interests and rights. The reforms and discussions ignited by the OHRP's review of the SUPPORT study have enriched the collective understanding of the ethical intricacies of conducting research with vulnerable groups, emphasizing the pivotal role of informed consent in maintaining the moral foundation of clinical research.

Changes in Research Practices and Informed Consent Procedures

In response to the SUPPORT study controversy, there has been a concerted effort to enhance the clarity and comprehensiveness of informed consent documents. This includes ensuring that potential risks and benefits are communicated more transparently, especially when research involves standard-of-care interventions that may carry unforeseen risks. Research institutions and IRBs have intensified their scrutiny of consent forms, emphasizing the need for lay language that is easily understandable to non-medical professionals. Additionally, there has been an increased focus on the process of informed consent, recognizing it as an ongoing dialogue between researchers and participants rather than a one-time transaction. Training programs for researchers now often include modules on ethical communication and how to effectively convey complex information about risks, benefits, and the nature of the study.

Influence on Ethical Guidelines and Regulations

The SUPPORT trial has prompted a reevaluation of ethical guidelines and regulations for clinical trials, leading to a broader discussion about how best to protect vulnerable populations in research. National and international bodies, including the NIH and the World Health Organization (WHO), have revisited their guidelines to address the ethical complexities highlighted by the SUPPORT controversy. This has involved clarifying the requirements for informed consent, particularly in comparative effectiveness research where the delineation of risks and benefits may be less clear. Efforts have been made to ensure that ethical guidelines are adaptable to the nuances of different types of research, without compromising the fundamental principles of respect for persons, beneficence, and justice.

Balancing Research Benefits with Participant Protection

The SUPPORT study controversy has underscored the critical need to balance the pursuit of scientific knowledge with the imperative to protect research participants. This balance is particularly delicate in studies involving vulnerable populations, where the potential for benefit must be weighed against the risk of harm. The controversy has led to a more nuanced understanding of risk in clinical research, recognizing that not all risks are quantifiable at the outset of a study. As a result, there is now a greater emphasis on monitoring and adaptive risk management throughout the study. This includes mechanisms for ongoing assessment of risks and benefits, enhanced communication with participants about new findings that may affect their willingness to continue, and the option for participants to withdraw without penalty.

The SUPPORT trial has served as a pivotal learning opportunity for the research community, highlighting the importance of ethical vigilance and the need for continuous improvement in the protection of human subjects. The changes implemented in the wake of the controversy reflect a collective commitment to upholding the highest ethical standards in clinical research. As the field evolves, the lessons learned from the SUPPORT trial will continue to inform best practices, ensuring that the rights and welfare of research participants are always at the forefront of scientific inquiry.

Legacy

The SUPPORT study, despite its controversies, has left a durable impression on neonatal research and the ethical standards governing clinical trials. Its impact reverberates through the ongoing efforts to refine the balance between advancing medical knowledge and ensuring the protection and rights of the most vulnerable research participants. The study has catalyzed a broader examination of ethical practices, particularly around the complexities of informed consent and risk communication in pediatric research.

The long-term impact of the SUPPORT study on neonatal research cannot be overstated. It has underscored the critical importance of ethical vigilance in studies involving premature infants, a population inherently at risk due to their medical fragility. The controversy surrounding the study prompted a reevaluation of how risks are communicated to parents and guardians, leading to more nuanced approaches that aim to convey complex information in a comprehensible manner. This shift has influenced not only neonatal research but also pediatric studies more broadly, encouraging a deeper engagement with ethical considerations from the study design phase through to the consent process.

Ongoing debates about risk communication and the consent process in pediatric research have been significantly shaped by the SUPPORT study. These debates often center on how to effectively balance the need for clear, understandable information with the complexity of the risks and benefits associated with participation in clinical research. The challenge lies in ensuring that parents and guardians are fully informed about the potential implications of a study without overwhelming them with technical details or unduly influencing their decision-making process. Examples of this ongoing dialogue can be found in the literature that critiques traditional consent forms and proposes innovative approaches, such as layered consent or the use of decision aids, to enhance understanding and facilitate informed decision-making.[9]

---

[9] Flory, J. and Emanuel, E. (2004) Interventions to improve research participants' understanding in informed consent for research: a systematic review. *JAMA.* 292(13):1593–1601. doi: 10.1001/jama.292.13.1593.

Furthermore, the SUPPORT study has played an indispensable role in fostering greater transparency and accountability in medical research. The public and professional scrutiny that followed the revelations about the study's consent process highlighted the need for research institutions and oversight bodies to operate with a higher degree of openness. This has led to calls for more public reporting of study protocols, consent forms, and IRB deliberations, as well as the outcomes of research studies, especially those involving vulnerable populations. The emphasis on transparency aims not only to protect participants but also to build public trust in the research process, a crucial element for the continued advancement of medical science.

The legacy of the SUPPORT study is a testament to the dynamic nature of ethical standards in clinical research. It serves as a reminder of the ongoing responsibility of researchers, ethicists, and regulatory bodies to adapt and respond to emerging ethical challenges. By continuing to engage with these complex issues, the research community can ensure that the pursuit of knowledge remains firmly grounded in the principles of respect, beneficence, and justice.

Conclusion

The SUPPORT study controversy has served as a turning point in the field of clinical research, offering profound ethical lessons and underscoring the necessity of rigorous ethical oversight. This episode has illuminated the complexities inherent in conducting research with vulnerable populations, particularly premature infants, and has highlighted the critical importance of informed consent as a cornerstone of ethical research practices.

One of the key ethical lessons learned from the SUPPORT study is the paramount importance of transparent and comprehensive risk communication within the informed consent process. The controversy revealed that even well-intentioned research aimed at improving outcomes for vulnerable populations could inadvertently compromise ethical standards if potential risks are not clearly communicated to participants or their surrogates. This lesson emphasizes that informed consent is not merely a regulatory requirement but a fundamental ethical obligation that respects the autonomy and dignity of research participants and their families. The SUPPORT study controversy has also reinforced the importance of rigorous ethical oversight in clinical research. It has demonstrated that ethical vigilance is essential not only in the planning and approval stages of research but throughout the conduct of the study. Oversight bodies, including Institutional Review Boards (IRBs) and regulatory agencies like the Office for OHRP, play a crucial role in ensuring that research protocols adhere to the highest ethical standards, especially when vulnerable populations are involved. This oversight is vital in maintaining public trust in the research enterprise and in safeguarding the welfare and rights of research participants.

Furthermore, the SUPPORT study has catalyzed a call for ongoing dialogue and continuous improvement in research ethics and informed consent practices. It has become evident that as medical science advances, so too must our ethical frameworks and practices evolve to address new challenges. There is a clear need for a dynamic and responsive approach to research ethics, one that fosters open dialogue among researchers, ethicists, regulatory bodies, and the public. Such dialogue is essential in developing innovative solutions to ethical dilemmas and in refining informed consent processes to better serve both the scientific community and research participants.

The SUPPORT study controversy has left an indelible mark on the landscape of clinical research ethics. It serves as a reminder of the ethical complexities of conducting research with vulnerable populations and the imperative of upholding the highest ethical standards. Moving forward, the lessons learned from this controversy should inspire a commitment to rigorous ethical oversight, continuous dialogue, and improvement in research practices. By embracing these principles, the research community can work to prevent similar controversies in the future and ensure that the pursuit of scientific knowledge proceeds with both integrity and respect for the dignity of all participants.

Chapter 11

Vulnerability Testing Program

The Cold War, a period of geopolitical tension between the United States and the Soviet Union and their respective allies, lasted from the end of World War II in 1945 until the dissolution of the Soviet Union in 1991. This era was characterized by a constant state of military and ideological competition, with both superpowers engaging in arms races to develop nuclear, chemical, and biological weapons. The fear of biological warfare became particularly pronounced due to its potential for mass casualties and the ability to disrupt societies without the immediate, visible destruction caused by nuclear or conventional weapons. Biological weapons were seen as a "poor man's atomic bomb," offering a way to inflict widespread harm at a lower cost and with fewer technological barriers than nuclear weapons.[1]

The U.S. government's vulnerability testing program during the Cold War, marked by the non-consensual exposure of its own civilians to biological and chemical agents, stands as a period fraught with ethical lapses and a profound lack of empathy for the unwitting subjects involved. Driven by the imperatives of national security and the specter of geopolitical tensions, these clandestine operations were conducted with a disconcerting disregard for the potential harm to individuals and communities. This chapter delves into the motivations, ethical dilemmas, and significant repercussions of these tests, shedding light on a troubling chapter of history that underscores the critical importance of ethical integrity, informed consent, and the protection of human dignity in scientific inquiry and

---

[1] https://nationalinterest.org/blog/buzz/introducing-poor-mans-atomic-bomb-biological-weapons-37437.

national defense strategies. As we explore the intricate web of decisions and actions that led to these experiments, the narrative reveals a glaring absence of foresight and empathy, prompting a reevaluation of the balance between safeguarding national interests and upholding the fundamental rights of individuals.

Brief Introduction to the U.S. Government's Decision to Conduct Vulnerability Testing on Civilians

In response to these fears and the perceived threat from the Soviet Union's advancements in biological warfare, the U.S. government initiated a series of secretive tests on its civilian population. Vulnerability testing is the practice of exposing environments, systems, or populations to agents (in this context, biological agents) under controlled conditions to assess potential vulnerabilities and the effectiveness of countermeasures. The rationale behind these tests was to assess the vulnerability of American cities and military installations to biological attacks and to understand the potential impact of such warfare on the nation's security. These tests, conducted without the knowledge or consent of the affected populations, involved the release of harmless and, in some cases, potentially harmful biological agents into the environment to simulate the effects of a biological attack.

Several historical events prompted concern about biological weapons in the US military and intelligence services. For example, the widespread use of chemical weapons during WWI demonstrated the potential for non-conventional warfare to inflict mass casualties and psychological terror. This experience laid the groundwork for considering other forms of non-conventional weapons, including biological agents. During World War II, the Japanese Imperial Army conducted extensive research and testing of biological weapons in occupied territories, particularly in China. Unit 731, a covert biological and chemical warfare research and development unit, carried out horrific experiments on prisoners, including vivisections and the deliberate infection with diseases, such as plague, anthrax, and cholera. Finally, the US intelligence services were acutely aware of the Soviet Union's advancements in military capabilities, including robust programs in nuclear, chemical, and biological weapons.[2,3]

The revelation of these activities underscored the potential lethality of biological warfare and the interest in developing similar capabilities as a deterrent.

The objective behind the U.S. government's testing on its civilians was multifaceted. Primarily, it sought to gauge the country's vulnerabilities to potential biological attacks, understanding that in the event of such warfare, preparedness could mean the difference between containment and catastrophe. This imperative was not merely speculative; it was a response to a world where the threat of mass destruction loomed large, and the boundaries of warfare were rapidly expanding beyond conventional means.

The context for these tests was a world stage fraught with competition for military superiority. The arms race was not just about stockpiling weapons but also about demonstrating technological prowess and strategic capabilities. In this environment, nuclear, chemical, and biological weapons each represented different facets of potential warfare, with biological weapons holding a particularly insidious appeal due to their ability to inflict widespread damage discreetly and with delayed onset.

Several U.S. organizations and their leaders played pivotal roles in orchestrating these tests. The Central Intelligence Agency (CIA), under the direction of figures like Sidney Gottlieb, spearheaded projects like MK-Ultra, which, while more famously known for its mind-control experiments, also delved into aspects of chemical and biological warfare. The U.S. Army Chemical Corps, operating out of facilities like Fort Detrick in Maryland, became a central hub for the development and testing of biological agents.

The rationale behind focusing on biological rather than solely on chemical or nuclear testing lies in the unique attributes of biological agents. Unlike nuclear weapons, which require significant resources to

---

[2] Miller, J., Engelberg, S. and Broad, W. (2001). *Germs: Biological Weapons and America's Secret War*. New York: Simon and Schuster.

[3] Leitenberg, M., Zilinskas, R.A. and Kuhn, J.H. (2012). *The Soviet Biological Weapons Program: A History*. Cambridge, MA: Harvard University Press.

develop and deploy, biological weapons could be produced more covertly and with potentially broader impacts on civilian populations. The insidious nature of the disease, with its ability to spread silently and widely before detection, presented a form of warfare that could destabilize societies without immediate recourse.

Chronology

The chronology of the United States government's secret vulnerability testing program, which spanned several decades during the Cold War, unfolds through a series of experiments that evolved in response to changing technologies, strategic priorities, and ethical considerations.[4] Starting in the early 1940s, the U.S. embarked on its formal biological warfare program, notably with the establishment of research facilities such as Camp Detrick, later known as Fort Detrick. This period marked the beginning of the United States' exploration into the potential of biological agents as weapons.

By 1950, the program had expanded to include tests on the American public, a notable example being Operation Sea-Spray. Operation Sea-Spray began on September 20th, 1950; the U.S. Navy initiated a covert biological warfare test in San Francisco, discreetly dispersing bacteria over the city.[5,6] For eight days, a vessel navigated the bay's perimeter, emitting large quantities of two distinct bacterium types. These were chosen for their supposed harmlessness and their ability to mimic the behavior of pathogens (i.e., a microorganism, including bacteria, viruses, or fungi, that can cause disease in humans, animals, or plants) that could be employed in a biological attack. Throughout this period, six simulated

---

[4] Human Experimentation: An Overview on Cold War Era Programs (Washington, D.C.: United States General Accounting Office, September 28, 1994), 3.

[5] Cole, L.A. (1990). *Clouds of Secrecy: The Army's Germ Warfare Tests Over Populated Areas*. Lanham, MD: Rowman and Littlefield.

[6] US Chemical Corps Biological Laboratories. *Biological Warfare Trials at San Francisco, California, 20-27 September 1950*. Special Report No. 142. Camp Detrick, Frederick, MD, January 22, 1951.

biological warfare assaults were executed: Bacillus globigii was used in four instances and Serratia marcescens in two.[7,8] The objective was to assess the vulnerability of a metropolitan area like San Francisco to an attack with biological weapons. From September 20 to September 27, these bacteria were released from a naval vessel positioned offshore. Monitoring devices placed at 43 different sites throughout the city indicated that the bacterial dispersion was widespread enough that virtually every one of the city's 800,000 inhabitants could have inhaled a minimum of 5,000 particles,[9] a quantity considered within the infective range for pathogens like anthrax.[10]

Following the experiment, on October 11, 1950, 11 individuals were admitted to Stanford Hospital in San Francisco with severe and uncommon urinary tract infections. Urinary tract infections with Serratia marcescens had never been seen before in the long history of the hospital. While ten of these patients eventually recovered, one patient, Edward J. Nevin, who had undergone prostate surgery recently, developed an Serratia marcescens infection of his heart valve and died three weeks later. The outbreak was deemed so unusual that it was documented in a medical journal by the Stanford medical team.[11] It was noted that no other hospitals in San Francisco reported a similar increase in such infections, and all 11 cases were linked to individuals who had undergone medical procedures, pointing to a nosocomial (hospital-acquired) origin of the infections. Additionally, there was a noted increase in pneumonia cases in the city following the dispersal of Serratia marcescens, though a direct link to the bacteria has not been definitively proven.

[7]Thompson, H. (2015). In 1950, the U.S. Released a Bioweapon in San Francisco. *Smithsonian Magazine*. Smithsonian Institution. ISSN 0037-7333 (Accessed 2/17/24).

[8]Kreston, R. (2015). Blood & Fog: The Military's Germ Warfare Tests in San Francisco. *Discover*. Archived from the original on 22 May 2020.

[9]Carlton, J. (2001). Of Microbes and Mock Attacks: Years Ago, The Military Sprayed Germs on U.S. Cities. *The Wall Street Journal* (Accessed 2/17/24).

[10]Coleman, M.E., Thran, B., Morse, S.S., Hugh-Jones, M. and Massulik, S. (2008). Inhalation anthrax: Dose response and risk analysis. *Biosecurity and Bioterrorism: Biodefense Strategy, Practice, and Science*. 6(2): 147–159. doi: 10.1089/bsp.2007.0066.

[11]Crockett, Z. (30 October 2014). How the U.S. Government Tested Biological Warfare on America. *Priceonomics* (Accessed 2/17/24).

This operation also had parallels in the United Kingdom, where, between 1971 and 1975, the bacterium, along with phenol and an anthrax simulant, was sprayed over south Dorset during the DICE trials conducted by U.S. and UK military scientists. A simulant is a substance or organism used in experiments to mimic the physical or biological properties of a real pathogen, without the associated risk of disease.

Critically, there was no indication that the Navy had informed local health authorities before conducting the experiment, leading to speculation among medical professionals about whether this operation could be linked to subsequent heart valve infections and severe infections among intravenous drug users in the 1960s and 1970s.

The 1960s saw further escalation with operations like "Operation Big City," where bacteria were released in the New York City subway system to study the potential for an attack on the city's underground transportation systems.[12,13] In February 1956, Operation Big City began with a Ford Mercury cruising the streets of Manhattan. The car was specially modified with an aerosol dispersal unit, which sprayed the bacteria Bacillus globulii into the streets of the city. Later, agents went into the subway system carrying attaché cases containing miniaturized aerosol devices which sprayed the bacteria on the platform before the onrushing trains. Ten years later, the US Army returned to repeat the experiment. This time, the agents carried glass bulbs filled with bacteria that were dropped in front of trains to test how far the bacteria would spread through the subway system. This era was characterized by a broadening of the scope of experiments, including both simulants and live agents to assess vulnerabilities and the effectiveness of biological agents under various conditions.

By 1969, the U.S. military had determined that biological warfare (BW) offered limited tactical advantage on the battlefield. In an era where nuclear weapons were the primary strategic focus, it was believed that the United States would unlikely resort to using biological weapons.

---

[12] US Army. A Study of the Vulnerability of Subway Passengers in New York City to Covert Action with Biological Agents. Miscellaneous Publication 25. Fort Detrick, Frederick, MD, January 1968.

[13] Cole, L.A. (2003). *The Anthrax Letters: A Medical Detective Story*. Washington, DC: National Academies Press.

Consequently, that same year, President Nixon declared the U.S.'s unilateral decision to renounce biological warfare and destroy its biological weapon stockpiles. This announcement was a pivotal moment in the history of biological warfare, signaling a shift in U.S. policy. The clear stance of the U.S. government against biological weapons paved the way for the negotiation of a comprehensive international treaty aimed at prohibiting biological warfare.

Despite this declaration, the research program continued and reached a peak of activity in the early 1970s, with a series of tests conducted in diverse environments, including urban areas, military bases, and other sensitive locations. These experiments were designed to assess the dispersion patterns of biological agents and the effectiveness of detection and decontamination methods. However, by the late 1970s and into the 1980s, the primacy of nuclear weapons, as well as the public and congressional scrutiny led to a significant decrease in the number of known tests. The focus shifted toward compliance with international treaties and the development of defensive measures against biological threats, marking a significant shift in the program's direction.

Throughout its duration, the U.S. government's vulnerability testing program was marked by a transition from initial explorations of biological warfare capabilities to operational testing in real-world scenarios and, ultimately, to a phase of public exposure and ethical reckoning. This shift was characterized by an increased emphasis on ethical standards and oversight, reflecting the complex balance between national security interests and the ethical obligations to protect citizens from undue harm. The program's evolution from the 1940s through the 1980s illustrates the changing landscape of military research and the growing awareness of the ethical implications of such testing on unsuspecting populations.

Key players and organizations

The United States' vulnerability testing program during the Cold War involved several key organizations and notable individuals whose roles were pivotal in the execution and oversight of these clandestine operations. Among the leading agencies, the CIA played a significant role, particularly through its MK-Ultra program, which is perhaps one of the most infamous examples of government-sponsored research into mind control and chemical warfare. Sidney Gottlieb, as the head of MK-Ultra, became a central figure in the CIA's efforts to develop techniques and substances for use in interrogation and espionage, with some aspects of the program veering into the territory of biological agents.

The Department of Defense (DoD) also had a crucial role in coordinating and funding research into biological and chemical weapons, acting as a bridge between political directives and military implementation. Within the DoD, the U.S. Army Chemical Corps emerged as a key player, tasked with the development and testing of chemical and biological warfare tactics. This corps conducted numerous field tests, including the dispersal of simulants and live agents to study potential military applications and the impacts of such weapons on enemy forces and civilian populations.

The leadership within these organizations, from program heads to key scientists, played a critical role in advancing the United States' capabilities in biological and chemical warfare. Figures like Gottlieb, with backgrounds in chemistry and espionage, brought a mix of scientific expertise and strategic thinking to programs that operated in the shadows, often bypassing the ethical considerations and oversight typically associated with research involving human subjects.

During the Cold War, the United States government's exploration into non-conventional warfare significantly emphasized biological weapons, distinguishing them from their chemical and nuclear counterparts. This focus was largely due to the unique advantages that biological agents offered, such as their stealth and the difficulty in detecting an attack, which could potentially allow for covert operations against adversaries without immediate attribution. Biological agents, by their nature, could be spread silently and invisibly, causing widespread panic and disorder before the source of the outbreak was identified. This aspect made them an attractive option for scenarios where deniability or surprise was a strategic priority.

The methodologies employed in the testing of these biological agents were diverse and often innovative, reflecting the experimental nature of the program. Open-air tests were a common approach, designed to simulate the release of biological agents in environments ranging from urban centers to rural settings. These tests aimed to understand how factors like wind, temperature, and population density affected the dispersion and impact of pathogens. Facilities like Fort Detrick in Maryland played a crucial role in this research, serving as the epicenter for the U.S. biological warfare program. Fort Detrick was equipped with state-of-the-art laboratories and testing grounds that allowed scientists to cultivate, store, and experiment with various biological agents under controlled conditions.

The agents used in these tests included a range of pathogens and chemicals, some of which were selected for their harmlessness as simulants to study dispersion patterns, while others had the potential to cause disease. Bacillus globigii, for example, was often used as a simulant because it is closely related to Bacillus anthracis, the bacterium that causes anthrax but is not harmful to humans.[14] Bacillus globigii spores are easy to detect and measure in environmental samples, facilitating the monitoring and analysis of experimental results. Its distinctive characteristics enable researchers to track its dispersion patterns and concentration levels accurately. Serratia marcescens, another bacterium employed in these tests, was chosen for its distinctive red pigment, which made it easy to track. Its physical size and behavior in aerosol form were considered like those of actual pathogens that might be used in biological warfare. This similarity helped researchers understand how a real biological attack might disperse and affect populations. Initially thought to be a harmless organism that decomposes organic material, Serratia marcescens is now understood to be a significant opportunistic pathogen.[15] It has a notable ability to cause infections in healthcare settings and to easily develop resistance to antibiotics. Its use led to unintended infections among the civilian population, highlighting the risks involved in even seemingly controlled experiments.

The choice of these agents reflected a calculated balance between the need to simulate realistic scenarios and the imperative to minimize harm to unwitting participants. However, the ethical implications of exposing

---

[14] Farrell, S, Halsall, H.B. and Heineman, W.R. (2005). Bacillus globigii bugbeads: A model simulant of a bacterial spore. *Anal Chem.* 77(2):549–555. doi: 10.1021/ac049156y.

[15] Yu, V.L. (1979). Serratia marcescens: Historical perspective and clinical review. *N Engl J Med.* 300:887–893.

populations to any level of risk without their consent were significant and have since been the subject of extensive debate and criticism.

Ethical analysis

The ethical implications of the U.S. government's vulnerability testing program during the Cold War, particularly the lack of informed consent from test subjects, have been the subject of intense scrutiny and debate. The core ethical issue at the heart of these experiments was the government's decision to expose civilians to biological and chemical agents without their knowledge or consent. This approach starkly contrasts with contemporary ethical standards in research, which prioritize informed consent and the protection of participants from harm.

The concept of informed consent, a fundamental principle in both medical and psychological research today, was largely disregarded during these tests. Participants were not informed of their involvement in the experiments, nor were they made aware of the potential risks. This omission deprived individuals of the opportunity to choose whether to accept those risks, violating their autonomy and rights. The immediate and long-term health effects of exposure to certain agents, although often downplayed or ignored at the time, have since been recognized as significant concerns. In some cases, such as the release of Serratia marcescens in San Francisco, the exposure led to infections and serious health complications for unsuspecting individuals. These outcomes highlight the potential for harm inherent in such experiments, raising profound ethical questions about the responsibility of researchers and government officials to protect the public from unnecessary risks.

Counter arguments

A counterargument to these ethical lapses starts with an analysis of the context where these programs were developed. The decision to conduct these tests was driven by national security imperatives. In the context of the Cold War, the United States faced unprecedented threats, including the possibility of biological warfare. Government and military officials argued that understanding the potential impact of biological agents on American cities and military installations was crucial for developing effective defense strategies. They noted that without real-world data on how biological agents disperse and affect populations, the nation would be ill-prepared to respond to an actual attack, potentially resulting in significant casualties and societal disruption.

At the time, both the United States and the Soviet Union were engaged in an arms race that extended beyond nuclear weapons to include chemical and biological warfare capabilities. Military officials contended that vulnerability testing was essential for staying ahead in this race, allowing the United States to develop countermeasures and potentially deter adversaries from considering biological attacks. The testing was seen as a necessary step in ensuring that the U.S. military and public health systems could effectively respond to and mitigate the effects of such warfare. This decision of the US Government to perform these vulnerability tests reflects the Cold War mentality, where national security concerns often took precedence over individual rights and ethical standards.

Officials also pointed to the ethical considerations and oversight mechanisms that were purportedly in place to minimize risk. They argued that the agents used in the tests were selected for their non-pathogenic nature to humans, under the belief that they posed minimal health risks. Furthermore, it was claimed that the testing was conducted under controlled conditions designed to ensure public safety. The intention was not to harm the population but to protect it by gaining knowledge critical for defense against biological threats. While these counterarguments provide insight into the rationale behind the vulnerability testing program, they also highlight the ethical dilemmas inherent in balancing national security with individual rights and public health.

Comparing these actions with contemporary ethical standards illuminates the evolution of research ethics over the past several decades. Modern guidelines, such as those outlined in the Declaration of Helsinki and enforced by institutional review boards (IRBs), emphasize the importance of informed consent, the minimization of harm, and the need for rigorous ethical oversight of research involving human subjects. These standards reflect a consensus within the scientific and medical communities that the rights and welfare of participants must be paramount in any research endeavor.

The legacy of the Cold War-era experiments has played a pivotal role in shaping current ethical guidelines for human subject research. The public and academic discourse surrounding these tests has underscored the necessity of balancing national security interests with individual rights and ethical considerations. The revelations of non-consensual experimentation contributed to a heightened awareness of the need for ethical oversight in research, leading to the establishment of more stringent ethical standards and procedures for protecting participants in both governmental and non-governmental research contexts.

In examining the ethical dimensions of the U.S. government's vulnerability testing program, it becomes clear that the lessons learned from this period have been instrumental in advancing the protection of human subjects in research. The emphasis on informed consent, ethical oversight, and the minimization of harm are now integral components of research ethics, serving as safeguards against the repetition of past abuses.

Revelations

The discovery of the U.S. government's vulnerability testing on civilians, which spanned several decades during the Cold War, came to light gradually, with significant revelations emerging in the 1970s and continuing into the 1990s as classified documents were declassified and investigative journalism uncovered the extent of these secret experiments. The public became increasingly aware of these tests through a combination of media reports, scholarly research, and the efforts of activists and victims seeking answers and accountability. One of the pivotal moments in this process was the publication of investigative pieces by journalists and the release of government documents under the Freedom of Information Act (FOIA), which detailed the scope and nature of the experiments conducted on unsuspecting American citizens.

The public reaction to these revelations was one of shock, anger, and disbelief. Many people were appalled to learn that the government had conducted experiments involving the release of chemical and biological agents in public spaces and on military personnel without informed consent. The media coverage played a crucial role in bringing these issues to the forefront of public consciousness, prompting widespread outcry and demanding accountability from those responsible. This coverage included detailed reports on the experiments themselves, the lack of consent from participants, and the potential health risks posed by the exposure to various agents.

The outcry led to congressional hearings, where lawmakers sought to understand the rationale behind the experiments, the extent of the testing, and the measures needed to prevent similar occurrences in the future.

The Church Committee, officially known as the United States Senate Select Committee to Study Governmental Operations with Respect to Intelligence Activities and chaired by Senator Frank Church, was one of the most notable. This committee, active from 1975 to 1976, delved into abuses by the CIA, NSA, FBI, and IRS. While its investigations were wide-ranging, covering various illegal intelligence activities, it also brought to light programs like MK-Ultra, where non-consensual testing and experimentation on humans were conducted, including the use of biological agents. Senator Church famously stated, "The United States must not adopt the tactics of the enemy. Means are as important as ends. Crisis makes it tempting to ignore the wise restraints that make men free. But each time we do so, each time the means we use are wrong, our inner strength, the strength of our values and our civilization, dies a little".[16]

Simultaneously, the House of Representatives formed the Pike Committee, officially the Select Committee on Intelligence and chaired by Congressman Otis G. Pike. Like the Church Committee, the Pike Committee, active during the same period, investigated covert military and intelligence operations. Although the Pike Committee's final report was not officially published due to national security concerns, leaked information contributed to the growing public awareness and concern over government practices.

These hearings were instrumental in shedding light on the government's actions, providing a platform for survivors and experts to testify about their experiences and the impact of the experiments. The hearings

---

[16] Church Committee Final Report, Book I, 1976.

contributed to a growing consensus on the need for stricter oversight of government research involving human subjects and the importance of ethical standards in conducting such research.

Survivors and individuals affected by the testing pursued justice through legal actions, seeking compensation and recognition of the harm they had suffered. These legal battles were often challenging, given the secrecy surrounding the experiments and the difficulty in proving causation between exposure and subsequent health issues. In 1981, the family of Edward J. Nevin took legal action against the federal government, claiming that negligence on the part of the government led to Nevin's death and resulted in financial and emotional distress for his widow due to medical expenses. However, the initial court decision was not in their favor, mainly because it was not conclusively proven that the bacteria released during the test caused Nevin's death. Undeterred, the Nevin family pursued their case through the appeals process, ultimately reaching the U.S. Supreme Court. The Supreme Court chose not to overturn the judgments of the lower court.[17]

Nevertheless, the persistence of survivors and their advocates brought attention to the individual stories behind the experiments, humanizing the broader ethical and legal debates. These efforts also contributed to the push for reforms, including the establishment of more robust ethical guidelines for human subject research and mechanisms for oversight and accountability in government-sponsored research.

The public and governmental response to the discovery of the U.S. government's vulnerability testing program reflects a critical juncture in the relationship between the state and its citizens, highlighting the tension between national security imperatives and the rights of individuals. The legacy of these experiments continues to influence public trust in government and the ethical standards governing research involving human subjects.

The revelation of the U.S. government's vulnerability testing on civilians during the Cold War catalyzed a seismic shift in policies governing

---

[17]LaFreniere, D. (2019). Forgiveness or Permission: How May the United States Government Conduct Experiments on the Public or in Public?. *Journal of Biosecurity, Biosafety, and Biodefense Law.* 10(1). doi: 10.1515/jbbbl-2019-0001.

human experimentation, fundamentally altering the landscape of research ethics and government accountability. In the wake of public outcry and congressional scrutiny, there was a concerted effort to establish more rigorous ethical review processes, enhance oversight mechanisms, and redefine the guidelines for human experimentation to prevent future abuses. These changes were aimed at restoring public trust in government research activities and ensuring that the rights and welfare of participants were protected.

One of the key outcomes of this period was the strengthening of ethical standards for human subject research. The National Research Act of 1974, for example, led to the creation of the National Commission for the Protection of Human Subjects of Biomedical and Behavioral Research, which was tasked with identifying the basic ethical principles that should underlie the conduct of biomedical and behavioral research involving human subjects. The commission's work culminated in the publication of the Belmont Report in 1979, which outlined fundamental ethical principles, such as respect for persons, beneficence, and justice. These principles became the cornerstone of ethical guidelines for research involving human subjects in the United States, influencing both governmental and non-governmental research endeavors.

Moreover, the establishment of IRBs became a mandatory requirement for any institution conducting research involving human subjects that received federal funding. IRBs were charged with reviewing research proposals to ensure that they met ethical standards, including the provision of informed consent, the minimization of risks to participants, and the equitable selection of subjects. This system of review and oversight represented a significant step forward in institutionalizing ethical considerations in the research process.

The legacy of the Cold War-era vulnerability testing extends beyond the realm of research ethics, impacting public trust in government and shaping policies regarding biological warfare preparedness. The disclosures of non-consensual experimentation contributed to a more cautious and skeptical public attitude toward government-led research initiatives, underscoring the importance of transparency, accountability, and ethical conduct. Additionally, these revelations prompted a reevaluation of policies related to biological warfare, with a greater emphasis on defensive measures and adherence to international treaties such as the Biological Weapons Convention (BWC), which the United States ratified in 1975. The BWC represents a global commitment to eliminating biological weapons, reflecting a shift toward prioritizing collective security and ethical considerations in the development and deployment of such capabilities.

The policy changes and legacy of the U.S. government's vulnerability testing program highlight the critical importance of ethical oversight and public accountability in the conduct of research involving human subjects. These developments have left an indelible mark on the principles and practices of research ethics, serving as a reminder of the potential consequences of neglecting the rights and welfare of individuals in the pursuit of scientific and national security objectives.

The exposure of these programs marked a pivotal moment in the history of research ethics and government accountability. This period of reckoning led to profound changes in how human experimentation was conducted and overseen, fundamentally reshaping the relationship between the state and its citizens in the context of scientific research.

In response to the public outcry and the ethical concerns raised by these tests, the U.S. government took significant steps to enhance the oversight and ethical review processes for human experimentation. One of the most notable outcomes was the establishment of the National Research Act of 1974, which laid the groundwork for the creation of the National Commission for the Protection of Human Subjects of Biomedical and Behavioral Research. This commission was instrumental in identifying the basic ethical principles that should guide the conduct of research involving human subjects, culminating in the publication of the Belmont Report in 1979. The Belmont Report articulated key ethical principles, including respect for persons, beneficence, and justice, which have since become the bedrock of ethical guidelines for human subject research in the United States.

The implementation of IRBs across research institutions represented another critical step in ensuring that research involving human subjects met stringent ethical standards. IRBs were tasked with reviewing research proposals to ensure they adhered to ethical guidelines, including informed consent, risk minimization, and equitable subject selection. This system of ethical oversight has become a cornerstone of research ethics, reflecting a commitment to protecting the rights and welfare of participants.

Furthermore, these events prompted a reevaluation of the United States' stance on biological warfare, contributing to a greater emphasis on defensive strategies and compliance with international agreements, such as the BWC. This international treaty prohibits the development, production, and stockpiling of biological and toxin weapons. Ratified by the United States in 1975, the BWC embodies a global commitment to the prohibition of biological weapons, reflecting a shift toward prioritizing ethical considerations and collective security in national and international policy.

These policy changes and the enduring legacy of the vulnerability testing program underscore the importance of ethical oversight and public accountability in research involving human subjects. They serve as a stark reminder of the potential consequences of neglecting the rights and welfare of individuals in the pursuit of scientific knowledge and national security objectives, highlighting the need for ongoing vigilance in upholding ethical standards in research.

Conclusion

The exploration of the U.S. government's vulnerability testing program during the Cold War, which involved the non-consensual exposure of civilians to biological and chemical agents, unveils a critical juncture in the interplay between national security, scientific inquiry, and ethical standards. This chapter has navigated through the complex motivations behind these tests, the ethical dilemmas they engendered, and the profound impact they had on public trust and policy reform. However, to fully appreciate the significance of these historical events, it is essential to draw explicit connections to contemporary issues in research ethics, national security, and public health, thereby underscoring the enduring relevance of this chapter's subject matter to today's readers.

In the realm of research ethics, the legacy of the Cold War-era testing programs shows the paramount importance of informed consent, transparency, and accountability in scientific research. These experiments, conducted under the veil of secrecy, highlight the potential for ethical lapses when the oversight of sensitive research is inadequate or when the perceived needs of national security overshadow the principles of informed consent and individual autonomy.

The establishment of IRBs and the formulation of guidelines that prioritize the protection of human subjects are direct responses to past abuses. Yet, as we navigate new frontiers in science and technology, from genetic engineering to artificial intelligence, these principles remain foundational, reminding us of the need for vigilance to prevent the recurrence of ethical transgressions.

Regarding national security, the historical context of these vulnerability tests highlights the challenges of balancing the imperatives of protecting national interests with ethical considerations. In today's interconnected world, where threats can emerge from both state and non-state actors and span the cyber and biological domains, the lessons learned from the Cold War are more pertinent than ever. The decision to renounce biological warfare and pursue international treaties like the BWC illustrates the potential for ethical leadership and cooperation in addressing security challenges. This approach remains critical as we confront contemporary threats and strive to prevent the militarization of scientific advancements.

The moral implications of the vulnerability testing program are profound, raising critical questions about the extent to which governments can go in experimenting with potentially dangerous substances on their populations without their consent. The lack of informed consent and the potential harm to participants not only violated ethical standards but also eroded public trust in government and scientific institutions. This period of history underscores the necessity of ethical vigilance and the importance of balancing scientific inquiry and national security interests with the rights and welfare of individuals.

In the sphere of public health, the unintended consequences of the vulnerability testing program — such as the infections caused by Serratia marcescens — underscore the potential public health risks associated with conducting research without adequate ethical oversight. Today, as we face global health challenges like pandemics and antibiotic resistance, the importance of ethical research practices that prioritize public safety and well-being cannot be overstated. The historical misuse of biological agents serves as a reminder of the need for robust public health policies and practices that are informed by ethical considerations and a commitment to protecting populations.

By drawing these connections, we not only enhance our understanding of the Cold War-era vulnerability testing program but also illuminate its relevance to contemporary debates and challenges in research ethics, national security, and public health. The lessons learned from this period offer valuable insights for navigating the ethical complexities of today's scientific and security landscapes, emphasizing the ongoing importance of ethical integrity, public accountability, and the protection of human dignity in all endeavors.

In reflecting on the vulnerability testing program, it becomes clear that historical accountability is not just about acknowledging past wrongs but also about learning from them to inform future actions. The importance of maintaining ethical standards in research, even — or especially — in times of perceived crisis, cannot be overstated. As society continues to navigate the challenges of scientific advancement and national security, the lessons learned from this period remain relevant, serving as a reminder of the need for a continuous commitment to ethical integrity and the protection of human dignity.

Further Reading

1. **"Clouds of Secrecy: The Army's Germ Warfare Tests Over Populated Areas" by Leonard A. Cole**
   - This book provides an in-depth look at the open-air tests conducted by the U.S. Army.
2. **"The Plutonium Files: America's Secret Medical Experiments in the Cold War" by Eileen Welsome**
   - Although focusing on radiation experiments, this Pulitzer Prize-winning book offers context on the broader scope of non-consensual government testing.
3. **"Undue Risk: Secret State Experiments on Humans" by Jonathan D. Moreno**
   - Moreno's work covers a range of government experiments, including those involving biological agents.

Chapter 12

Looking Ahead: Safeguarding the Future of Medical Research

This chapter envisions a future where medical research is conducted within a framework that prioritizes ethics and transparency. It reflects on the lessons learned from past abuses in medical research, emphasizing the need for a shift toward more responsible and respectful research practices. This chapter sets the stage for a discussion on actionable recommendations for various stakeholders in the medical research community.

Vision for a More Ethical and Transparent Research Environment

The cornerstone of ethical medical research lies in its adherence to core ethical principles: respect for persons, beneficence, and justice. These principles, as articulated in seminal documents like the Belmont Report, provide a moral framework that should guide every aspect of medical research.

- Respect for persons involves acknowledging the autonomy of individuals and protecting those with diminished autonomy. In practice, this principle mandates informed consent, ensuring participants are fully aware of the research's nature, risks, and benefits before participating.
- Beneficence requires that researchers minimize harm and maximize benefits, not only for participants but also for society at large. This

principle demands a thorough risk–benefit analysis before initiating studies, ensuring that the potential benefits justify any risks.
- Justice entails distributing the benefits and burdens of research fairly. Research should not disproportionately target or exclude specific groups, particularly those vulnerable to exploitation or with limited access to healthcare benefits.

Operationalizing these principles in research settings requires robust ethical review processes, such as those conducted by Institutional Review Boards (IRBs), and ongoing ethical education for researchers to navigate complex ethical dilemmas that arise during studies.

Transparency is pivotal at all stages of medical research, from conceptualization and design through to the dissemination of results. It fosters trust, facilitates peer review, and encourages the application of findings in clinical practice:

- **Open Access to Research Protocols and Findings**: Making research protocols and results publicly accessible ensures that the scientific community and the public can evaluate the validity and reliability of findings. This can be achieved through open-access publications and registries for clinical trials, where methodologies and data are available for scrutiny.
- **Transparent Reporting**: Adhering to guidelines such as the CONSORT statement for clinical trials ensures that studies are reported with clarity, completeness, and transparency, allowing for the reproducibility of research and the verification of results.

The ethical conduct of research is deeply influenced by the institutional culture within which it occurs. Creating an environment that promotes ethical practices and holds individuals accountable for misconduct is essential for safeguarding the integrity of medical research:

- **Ethical Leadership**: Institutions should demonstrate a commitment to ethics from the top down. Leaders in research institutions and academic centers must embody ethical principles in their decision-making and interactions, setting a standard for others to follow.

- **Training and Resources**: Providing researchers and staff with ongoing training in research ethics and access to resources for ethical decision-making supports a culture of integrity. This includes training in the responsible conduct of research, data management practices, and the ethical implications of emerging technologies.
- **Mechanisms for Reporting and Addressing Misconduct**: Establishing clear, accessible channels for reporting ethical concerns or misconduct without fear of retaliation is crucial. Institutions must have procedures in place to investigate allegations thoroughly and take appropriate action to correct and prevent future ethical breaches.

By embedding these ethical foundations into the fabric of medical research, we can aspire to a future where research not only advances knowledge and improves patient care but does so with the highest ethical standards, ensuring the respect, safety, and fairness owed to all participants and society at large.

Recommendations for Physicians, Researchers, and Policymakers

In the realm of medical research and practice, the responsibility to uphold ethical standards extends beyond adherence to regulations; it is a commitment to the dignity and welfare of patients and research participants. For physicians and researchers, this commitment necessitates a dedication to continuous ethical training and education, as well as active engagement in ethical discourse.

Comprehensive ethics training for medical researchers and physicians is paramount. Such training should not only cover the foundational principles of research ethics, including respect for autonomy, beneficence, and justice, but also delve into the practical aspects of obtaining informed consent and safeguarding the interests of vulnerable populations. This education should not be viewed as a one-time requirement but as an ongoing process, evolving with the advancements in medical science and the complexities of modern healthcare. By advocating for and participating in continuous ethical education, medical professionals can stay abreast of emerging ethical challenges and best practices for addressing them.

Moreover, the cultivation of a community that values ethical considerations as central to research excellence is crucial. Physicians and researchers should be encouraged to actively participate in ethical discussions and decision-making processes. This can be facilitated through forums, workshops, and conferences dedicated to exploring ethical dilemmas in medical research and practice. Such platforms not only foster a culture of ethical vigilance but also promote the exchange of ideas and experiences, enriching the collective understanding of ethical best practices.

Engagement in ethical discourse also extends to the publication and peer review process, where researchers and physicians can contribute to the ethical integrity of scientific literature by ensuring that studies are reported transparently and responsibly. By advocating for ethical standards in research and clinical practice, and by actively participating in the broader ethical discourse, medical professionals can lead by example, inspiring a culture of ethical excellence in the medical community.

This approach to ethical training and engagement not only enhances the quality and integrity of medical research but also strengthens public trust in the medical profession. It underscores the medical community's commitment to conducting research and providing care that respects individual rights and promotes the well-being of society as a whole.

The stewardship of medical research ethics and the promotion of transparency are critical responsibilities that fall to policymakers. They are tasked with developing and enforcing comprehensive regulatory frameworks to ensure research adheres to the highest ethical standards, protects participant rights, and maintains transparency throughout the research process. A prime example of such ethical regulation is the Declaration of Helsinki, which globally sets the benchmark for conducting ethical medical research. In the United States, the Clinical Trials Registry exemplifies a commitment to transparency, mandating the registration and results reporting of clinical trials, thereby enhancing accountability in medical research.

Policymakers are also crucial in creating an environment conducive to ethical research. This role extends beyond merely setting standards; it involves ensuring adequate funding and support for research that not only meets ethical guidelines but also addresses pressing medical needs, such as research into rare diseases. These conditions, often overlooked due to their lack of commercial viability, represent a significant public health concern. By allocating resources to such underfunded areas, policymakers can democratize the benefits of medical research, ensuring equitable access across society.

Public–private partnerships stand out as a successful model for advancing ethical research, particularly in tackling diseases like tuberculosis and HIV/AIDS. These collaborations between government health agencies and pharmaceutical companies combine the strengths of both sectors, fostering the development of innovative treatments while adhering to ethical standards. Such partnerships highlight the potential for collective efforts to overcome barriers to access and affordability, ensuring that advancements in medical research benefit all segments of the population.

To further clarify the role of policymakers in the ethical oversight of medical research, it is essential to consider the challenges and opportunities inherent in this process. Recent legislative efforts, such as the 21st Century Cures Act in the United States, aim to streamline the development and delivery of new treatments while maintaining ethical oversight. Internationally, guidelines like those proposed by the World Health Organization on the ethical conduct of human genome editing underscore the global consensus on the need for a balanced approach that fosters innovation while safeguarding ethical principles.

Addressing these challenges requires a nuanced understanding of the dynamic landscape of medical research, where rapid advancements in technology and treatment modalities must be matched by equally adaptive regulatory frameworks. Policymakers must navigate these complexities, ensuring that regulations facilitate innovation without compromising ethical standards. Through informed legislation, targeted funding, and strategic collaborations, policymakers can steer medical research toward outcomes that not only advance scientific knowledge but do so with an unwavering commitment to ethics, equity, and the public good.

The importance of engaging the public in understanding the ethical dimensions of medical research cannot be overstated, as it lays the foundation for a relationship based on transparency and trust between the research community and the broader society. To effectively foster this understanding, a multifaceted approach is necessary, encompassing collaborations with media, educational initiatives, and direct public involvement in ethical decision-making.

Collaborations with media outlets serve as a vital conduit for conveying accurate and accessible information about medical research to the public. By demystifying the scientific and ethical complexities of research, these partnerships can illuminate the significance of ethical practices in research and underscore the societal implications of scientific advancements. For example, a series of articles or broadcasts that explain the ethical considerations behind clinical trials can enlighten the public on why certain protocols are necessary for safeguarding participant welfare.

Educational institutions also play a pivotal role in cultivating a society that is knowledgeable about medical research ethics. Through the development of curricula that incorporate ethical discussions into science education and the organization of public lectures that address contemporary issues in medical research, educational institutions can equip individuals with the critical thinking skills needed to navigate and contribute to ethical debates in research.

Direct public involvement in the ethical oversight of research represents a crucial strategy for democratizing the research process. Patient advisory panels and public consultations create avenues for incorporating diverse perspectives into research governance, particularly from groups that have historically been excluded from these conversations. The implementation of community advisory boards in clinical trials, especially those conducted within vulnerable communities, exemplifies how such mechanisms can foster a reciprocal relationship between researchers and the communities they study. These boards enable community members to voice their concerns and preferences, ensuring that research initiatives are aligned with the community's needs and ethical standards.

In the wake of scandals or controversies related to research practices, rebuilding public trust becomes paramount. Initiatives such as open days at research facilities, where the public can interact with researchers and gain insights into the research process, and participatory workshops on research ethics, play a significant role in this regard. Additionally, the inclusion of lay members in national ethics committees can further enhance the transparency and accountability of research, demonstrating a commitment to incorporating public values into research ethics.

By adopting these strategies, the research community can effectively bridge the divide between scientific innovation and societal values, ensuring that the pursuit of knowledge progresses hand in hand with ethical integrity and public engagement. This approach not only enriches the research process but also ensures that advancements in medical science are achieved with the informed support and understanding of the society they aim to benefit.

Ethical Challenges in Vulnerable Populations and Genetic Research

Research involving vulnerable populations necessitates a framework that goes beyond standard ethical considerations to address the unique risks and needs of these groups. For instance, studies involving children should not only ensure informed consent through guardians but also assent from the children themselves, as appropriate to their age and understanding. The ethical principle of beneficence must be rigorously applied to minimize risks and maximize potential benefits for these participants. An example of ethical research in vulnerable populations can be found in pediatric oncology trials, where the potential benefits of experimental treatments are carefully weighed against the risks, and special attention is given to the child's and family's understanding of the study.[1]

In genetic research, the privacy concerns are exemplified by the use of genetic data in criminal investigations, such as in the Golden State Killer case. This incident raised questions about the ethical use of genetic databases and the consent of individuals who submit their DNA for genealogical purposes, not anticipating law enforcement access. The ethical debate centers around the balance between solving crimes and protecting individuals' privacy rights. Scholars have discussed these issues

---

[1]American Academy of Pediatrics, Committee on Bioethics, 2019 https://publications. aap.org/collection/528/Committee-on-Bioethics?autologincheck=redirected (Accessed 2/19/24).

extensively, suggesting the need for clear consent processes and privacy protections for genetic data.[2]

Digital Health, AI, and Genomics: Navigating New Ethical Frontiers

In the realm of digital health, technologies like wearable devices and telehealth platforms are collecting vast amounts of personal health data. While these developments hold the promise of significant improvements in healthcare outcomes, they also introduce new ethical challenges that could potentially harm patients if not carefully managed.

The ethical challenge arises in safeguarding this data against unauthorized access or breaches, which could compromise patient privacy. An example of potential harm is the unauthorized use of sensitive health data, leading to privacy violations or even discrimination in employment or insurance. The case of Strava, a fitness tracking app, updated an online map showing the routes of over a billion workouts in 2017. In doing so, they exposed the locations of secret US military bases in Turkey, Syria, and Yemen.[3] This underscores the unintended consequences of collecting and sharing personal data.[4]

Artificial intelligence, particularly in diagnostics and treatment algorithms, relies on large datasets to learn and make predictions. The ethical concern here is twofold: the risk of algorithmic bias and the opacity of AI decision-making processes. For instance, if the data used to train AI systems lack diversity, the resulting algorithms could perpetuate biases, leading to disparities in healthcare outcomes for underrepresented groups.

---

[2]Erlich, Y., Shor, T., Pe'er, I. and Carmi, S. (2018). Identity inference of genomic data using long-range familial searches. *Science*. 362(6415):690–694. doi: 10.1126/science. aau4832. Epub 2018 Oct 11.

[3] https://www.businessinsider.com/secret-us-military-bases-world-strava-heat-map-operational-security-compromised-fitness-trackers-2018-1#:~:text=An%20interactive%20heat%20map%20from,stands%20the%20most%20to%20lose (Accessed 2/19/24).

[4]Rosenberg, M., Confessore, N. and Cadwalladr, C. (2018). *How Trump Consultants Exploited the Facebook Data of Millions*. The New York Times.

A notable case is the use of AI in predicting patient care needs, where an algorithm was found to be biased against black patients, assigning them lower risk scores than white patients with similar conditions.[5]

Additionally, the "black box" nature of some AI systems can obscure the rationale behind clinical decisions, challenging the principle of informed consent and potentially leading to mistrust or harm if incorrect diagnoses or treatments are suggested.

Genomic research, with its capacity to unlock personalized medicine, also navigates complex ethical waters. The collection and analysis of genetic information pose risks related to consent, privacy, and the potential for genetic discrimination. A specific concern is the long-term storage and use of genetic data, which could be accessed by third parties without the individual's consent, leading to discrimination based on genetic predispositions. Moreover, the implications of genetic findings can extend beyond the individual to affect family members, raising questions about consent and the sharing of potentially sensitive information.

The HeLa cells' controversy, where Henrietta Lacks' cells were used for research without her or her family's consent, illustrates the ethical issues surrounding consent and the use of biological materials for research.[6]

Globalization of Clinical Trials

The globalization of clinical trials, especially in low- and middle-income countries, raises ethical concerns about exploitation and equity. Controversies have arisen over trials for HIV/AIDS medications and vaccines, where the adequacy of informed consent was questioned. And the selection of participant populations for clinical trials raised ethical questions. An example is the controversy over clinical trials conducted in Africa. These trials were conducted without informed consent or

---

[5] Obermeyer, Z., Powers, B., Vogeli, C. and Mullainathan, S. (2019). Dissecting racial bias in an algorithm used to manage the health of populations. *Science*. 66(6464):447–453. doi: 10.1126/science.aax2342.

[6] Skloot, R. (2010). *The Immortal Life of Henrietta Lacks*. Crown Publishing Group.

understanding of the research by participants, leading to allegations of exploitation.[7]

The Future of Ethical Oversight

The partnership between DeepMind and the UK's National Health Service (NHS), where patient data were used to develop healthcare applications, exemplifies the ethical challenges at the intersection of technology and healthcare. In 2015, the Royal Free NHS Foundation Trust provided personal data of approximately 1.6 million patients to Google's Deep Mind as part of clinical safety tests of a new application 'Streams'. The application is designed to provide an alert, diagnosis, and detection system for acute kidney injury. On July 3, 2017, the Information Commissioner's Office (ICO) announced that the Royal Free NHS Foundation Trust had failed to comply with the Data Protection Act 1998.[8] The ICO ruled that the trust had breached the law when it provided patient details to Google's DeepMind as part of a 2015 deal.

The ICO said that patients would not have reasonably expected their information to have been used in this way, and the trust could and should have been far more transparent with patients. The ICO also found several shortcomings in how the data was handled, including that patients were not adequately informed.

The investigation by the UK's Information Commissioner's Office highlights the need for stringent data protection measures and transparency in the use of health data for research (ICO, 2017).[9]

These examples underscore the need for a robust ethical framework that addresses the unique challenges posed by emerging technologies in human research. Protecting patients from harm requires not only rigorous

---

[7] Petryna, A. (2009). *When Experiments Travel: Clinical Trials and the Global Search for Human Subjects*. Princeton University Press.

[8] https://hsfnotes.com/data/2017/07/08/google-deepmind-trial-failed-to-comply-with-data-protection-law/#:~:text=On%203%20July%202017%20the,patient%20details%20to%20Google's%20DeepMind (Accessed 2/19/24).

[9] https://www.digitalhealth.net/2016/05/ico-aware-of-google-deepmind-and-royal-free-app-concerns/ (Accessed 5/17/24).

data protection measures and transparency in AI decision-making but also careful consideration of the broader societal implications of genomic research. As we navigate this new frontier, the ethical principles of respect for persons, beneficence, and justice must guide our approach, ensuring that technological advancements enhance, rather than compromise, patient welfare, and equity in healthcare.

Conclusion

The path to ethical and transparent medical research demands collaboration from all involved — physicians, researchers, policymakers, and the public. Physicians and researchers must weave ethical principles into their work, continuously educating themselves and engaging in ethical discourse. Policymakers have the crucial role of creating and enforcing regulations that uphold the highest ethical standards, directing resources toward research that fills critical health gaps. The public, by staying informed and involved, plays a key role in ensuring research aligns with societal values and ethical standards, helping restore trust in the research community. Successful models of community engagement and international cooperation highlight the benefits of inclusive research approaches. Embracing ethical integrity across the board helps the medical research community learn from past errors, ensuring future endeavors respect human dignity and contribute positively to society. This united effort toward ethical research promises advancements in healthcare that are both scientifically robust and morally sound.

Conclusion

"The best interest of the patient is the only interest to be considered ..."

William J. Mayo, MD[1]

As we conclude our exploration into the somber history of patient abuse in medical research, we have navigated through the shadows cast by the pursuit of knowledge without ethical restraint. The narratives from the Tuskegee Syphilis Study to the unsettling experiments of MK-Ultra serve as stark reminders of the critical need to anchor medical research in ethical principles. These historical episodes reveal the fragility of ethical standards when overshadowed by scientific ambition and underscore the resilience of human dignity under the protection of rigorous ethical oversight. Yet, as we stand at the frontier of new scientific breakthroughs, from the intricacies of genomic editing to the vast potential of artificial intelligence in healthcare, the lessons gleaned from these past transgressions must steer us toward a proactive engagement with the ethical challenges that lie ahead.

To effectively meet these challenges, a comprehensive strategy is essential — one that encompasses continuous education in ethics for researchers and physicians, the establishment of robust regulatory frameworks, and the promotion of meaningful public engagement.

---

[1] Commencement Address, Rush Medical College, University of Chicago, June 15, 1910. *Collected Papers of St. Mary's Hospital, Mayo Clinic.* 1910; 2:557–566.

For researchers and medical professionals, ethics should transcend being a mere academic requirement and evolve into a continuous, reflective practice that keeps pace with scientific advancements. Policymakers are tasked with the crucial role of forming independent oversight bodies capable of enforcing ethical compliance, bridging the gap between policy and practice. Moreover, the creation of a global registry for all human research endeavors, mirroring the Clinical Trials Registry but broader in scope, would significantly enhance transparency and accountability.

Addressing the ethical quandaries presented by emerging technologies such as CRISPR and AI necessitates a nuanced understanding of their implications for patient rights and privacy. The ethical frameworks guiding our approach must be adaptable, capable of addressing issues like consent in the era of genomic data and ensuring equitable access to AI-driven healthcare innovations. Despite progress in legal and policy reforms, notable gaps persist, largely due to the rapid pace of technological advancements outstripping legislative responses. Bridging these gaps requires not only comprehensive regulation but also international cooperation to ensure that ethical standards in medical research are universally upheld.

Public engagement plays a pivotal role in ethical medical research, challenging us to find innovative ways to communicate and educate. Overcoming barriers such as mistrust, language differences, and varying levels of health literacy calls for targeted outreach programs and the leveraging of digital platforms to ensure that diverse voices contribute to ethical decision-making. This engagement is vital for rebuilding trust following research-related scandals and for ensuring that research agendas align with societal values and needs.

Reflecting on our collective moral responsibilities, it is evident that the duty to promote ethical research extends beyond the confines of the research community to encompass all of society. By participating in public discourse on medical ethics, advocating for transparent and accountable research practices, and supporting policies that prioritize patient rights, we can contribute to a future where medical research is synonymous with ethical integrity.

Looking forward, the vision for a more ethical and transparent research environment presents both a challenge and an opportunity. It is a call to action for physicians, researchers, policymakers, and the public to unite in the pursuit of scientific advancement that respects human dignity and promotes the greater good. Let this book serve not only as a reflection on the past but also as a blueprint for preventing future ethical transgressions in medical research. By embracing education, enhancing regulatory frameworks, fostering public engagement, and encouraging global cooperation, we can aspire to a future where medical research advances not just in scientific knowledge but in ethical wisdom as well. This commitment to ethical integrity in medical research is our path forward, ensuring that the legacy of medical research is defined by its capacity to heal, innovate, and uplift humanity in an ethically sound manner.

Index

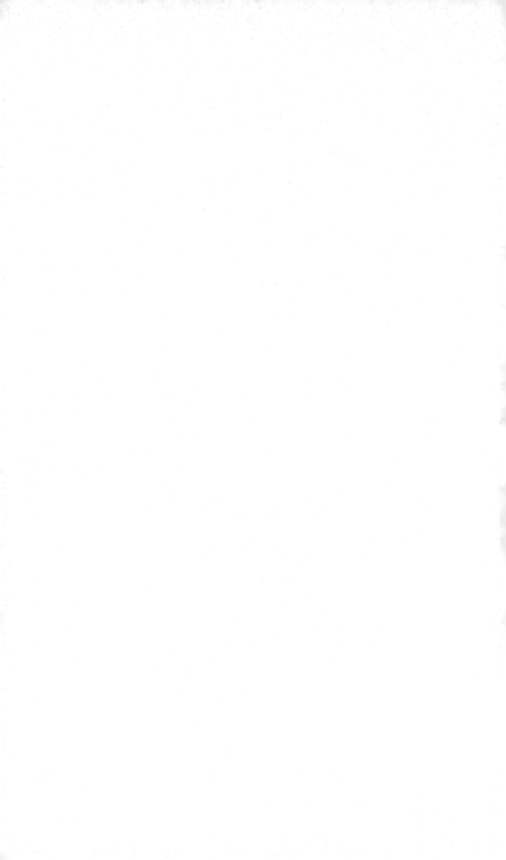

Printed in the United States
by Baker & Taylor Publisher Services